TIRED OF THE ENDLESS SUBTRACTING AND
CALCULATING?

CONFUSED AND DISCOURAGED BY TRYING TO
DECIPHER FOOD LABEL INFORMATION?

STYMIED BY RESTAURANT MENUS?

CONCERNED OVER WHAT FOODS TO BUY AND
PREPARE THAT WILL BEST SUIT YOUR NEW
LOW-CARB LIFESTYLE?

NET CARB COUNTER

lays out all the necessary information for you in a
convenient, easy-to-use-and-understand format.

PLUS:

- Up-to-date health information
- How to determine your personal Body Mass
  Index
- The Glycemic Index—what it is and why it's
  important
- The calorie, protein, and fat content—as well
  as net carbs—in the foods you eat every day

AND MUCH MORE

D0829252

NET
CARB
COUNTER

SHEILA BUFF

AVON BOOKS
An Imprint of HarperCollinsPublishers

This book contains advice and information relating to health care. It is not intended to replace medical advice and should be used to supplement rather than replace regular care by your doctor. It is recommended that you seek your physician's advice before embarking on any medical program or treatment. All efforts have been made to assure the accuracy of the information contained in this book as of the date of publication. The publisher and the author disclaim liability for any medical outcomes that may occur as a result of applying the methods suggested in this book.

AVON BOOKS
An Imprint of HarperCollins*Publishers*
10 East 53rd Street
New York, New York 10022-5299

Copyright © 2005 by Sheila Buff
ISBN: 0-06-082152-3
www.avonbooks.com

First Avon Books paperback printing: July 2005

Avon Trademark Reg. U.S. Pat. Off. and in Other Countries, Marca Registrada, Hecho en U.S.A.
HarperCollins ® is a registered trademark of HarperCollins Publishers Inc.

Printed in the U.S.A.

10 9 8 7 6 5 4 3

CONTENTS

NET CARB FOOD TABLES

INTRODUCTION

Today, around the country and around the world, millions of people are losing weight and improving their health while eating nutritious, varied, and delicious food. And they're doing all this without hunger pangs, food cravings, or feelings of deprivation.

What's their secret? They've discovered low-carb dieting.

Even better, they've discovered how easy it is to get rid of the low-quality carbohydrates in their diet and replace them with delicious, varied foods—foods that are low in carbs but high in nutrition. Gone are the doughnuts, french fries, cookies, and chips. In their place are vegetables, whole grains, fruit, good fats, high-quality protein, and other nutrient-rich foods. The changes are simple to make and easy to stick with—and for most people they lead to weight loss.

Low-carb dieting is usually very safe and effective. The more you know about it, the better you can stick with a low-carb diet and keep the weight off.

ONE

Low-Carb Concepts

Everybody's talking about carbohydrates, but what are they? And why does cutting back on them in your diet help you lose weight?

Let's start by understanding what carbohydrates are. Put simply, carbohydrates are the starchy or sugary part of foods. They're made up of long chains of molecules of carbon, hydrogen, and oxygen. Shorter, simpler chains of carbohydrates are sugars such as sucrose (table sugar), fructose (the sugar found in fruit), and glucose (the sugar that your body uses for fuel). Longer chains of carbohydrates are starchier and don't taste sweet—these complex carbs are found in plant foods such as vegetables, beans, and grains. When you eat complex carbohydrates, your body quickly breaks them down into simpler sugars. (An easy way to prove this to yourself is to put a piece of plain white bread into your mouth and hold it there. You'll notice a slight sweet taste as digestive enzymes in your saliva begin to convert the bread into glucose.)

So, when your body digests carbohydrates, it converts them into glucose, which then enters your bloodstream. To carry the glucose from your blood into your cells, your body releases the hormone insulin. So far, so good—but if you eat a diet high in carbs, the system doesn't work all that smoothly. Digesting the carbs puts a lot of extra glucose into your blood, which in turn mean you have to produce a lot of insulin to carry it into your cells. But if your cells have all the fuel they need for the moment, the extra glucose can't go into them. Instead, the insulin carries it off to be stored—mostly as body fat.

For many people, eating a lot of refined carbohydrates—foods such as white bread, snack foods, chips, french fries, sugary soft drinks, and all the other processed foods that take up so large a part of the typical diet—does more than just make them gain weight. The simple sugars in refined carbs hit your bloodstream soon after you eat. Your body puts out a surge of insulin to deal with all that glucose, and you get a quick surge of energy. But for a lot of people, that insulin surge works all too well—it clears away so much of the extra sugar that the energy surge is followed by an energy crash and feelings of hunger. What happens then? You reach for a candy bar or cookie for some more quick energy. It's a cycle of energy ebbs and flows that leads almost inevitably to putting on weight.

Here's where the low-carb approach comes in. First, you eliminate those refined carbohydrates from your diet and replace them with nutritionally dense whole foods. That means you're now eating a much healthier diet, because you've eliminated highly processed sugary or starchy foods that have little or no nutritional value. These foods can be high in salt and dangerous trans fats (you'll learn more about those later in this book), and they tend to crowd out more nutritious foods from your diet. Second, your blood sugar stays on a more even keel, giving you steady energy throughout the day. And third, you lose weight if you need to, because when you take away the carbs, your body burns fat for fuel instead.

HOW LOW IS LOW?

If you need to lose weight, cutting carbs is almost certain to help. The approach works because you're replacing low-quality, high-calorie refined carbs with small amounts of high-quality carbs, along with plenty of fresh vegetables and other good low-carb foods, good fats, and high-quality protein. But how low do you need to go?

If you follow the approach taken by two of the leading low-carb diet doctors—the late Dr. Robert C. Atkins and Dr. Arthur Agatston of South Beach Diet fame—you'll start off by cutting your net carb count down to just 20 grams a day for the first two or three weeks. (Net carbs are the carbohydrates in a food minus the fiber—Chapter Two of this book will explain this more.) After that, you'll slowly increase your daily carbohydrate intake. To continue losing weight, you'll probably have to keep your net carb count to under 60 grams a day. How your body responds to carbs is very individual, however. Some people will stop losing weight or even gain at just 40 grams of net carbs a day, while others can keep losing or stay at a steady weight at up to 100 or even 120 grams a day. Generally speaking, low-carbing means you're sticking to under 120 net carb grams a day (up to 150 grams a day for very active people), but you'll probably have to experiment a bit to find the level that's best for you.

To put all this in perspective, take a look at the typical carbohydrate counts for some commonly eaten foods:

1 slice white bread = 12 grams
8 ounces orange juice = 27 grams
5 Oreo® cookies = 55 grams
1 medium banana = 28 grams
1 12-ounce can cola soda = 27 grams
10 french fries = 16 grams

Is it any surprise that the average person takes in any-where from 200 to 300 grams of carbohydrates a day? (When looking at these numbers, it helps to remember that there are roughly 15 grams in a tablespoon and about 30 grams in an ounce.) Unfortunately, many of those carb grams come from sugary or salty snacks that are high in calories but low in nutrition. In fact, Americans today get about one-third of their daily calories from snack foods. It's no wonder over half of all Americans today are overweight. By cutting back on carbs, you're almost automatically cut-ting back on the lowest-quality foods in your diet and sub-stituting better foods such as fresh vegetables and protein.

CHOOSING THE RIGHT PROTEIN

When you go on a low-carb diet, all you eat is bacon, steak, and eggs, right? Absolutely not. While those foods can cer-tainly be an enjoyable part of a low-carb diet, they're just a part—and you don't have to eat them at all if you don't want to. Many vegetarians have successfully lost weight on low-carb diets.

Protein is an important part of low-carb dieting, however. Especially when it's combined with dietary fat, protein does a lot to help you feel satisfied by your food and to keep you satisfied for longer. When you have to limit your protein portions, as low-calorie diets recommend, you end up feel-ing hungry soon after a meal.

Your body needs adequate protein to function properly. How much? On average, you require about 7 ounces of high-quality protein a day. Any less and you're not really getting adequate nutrition. High-quality protein is any pro-tein that's complete—that is, it contains all eight essential amino acids. In general, that means animal protein from meat, poultry, eggs, fish, seafood, and dairy products. Vegetable protein sources, such as tofu, tend to be on the low side for one or more amino acids, but you can make up the difference by making smart food combinations—another reason it's quite possible to go low-carb without meat.

VARIETY AND VEGETABLES

The low-carb approach means you eat a wide variety of healthy foods. In fact, if you start low-carbing, you'll probably start eating more vegetables than you've ever eaten before. Even on the strictest part of the Atkins or South Beach diet, for instance, when net carbs are limited to 20 grams a day, that still works out to four cups of salad greens and a substantial portion of some other vegetable such as cauliflower. Those portions aren't optional—they're *essential* to the low-carb approach. At least five servings of vegetables (preferably more) become a regular part of your daily diet forever. One interesting thing about low-carb dieting is the way even people who have always hated eating their veggies start to really like them. They discover a new world of interesting flavors and textures based on real food, not packaged junk.

THE GOOD CARBS

On any low-carb diet, you still get to eat some carbohydrates even in the most restrictive phase. In the later stages you gradually add back more carbs, but you're always told to make them "good" carbs. It's pretty clear you can't blow your extra carb allowance on potato chips, but what can you add back? A surprising number of great foods, as long as you keep to small portions and stay aware of how your choices will affect your daily net carb count.

In general, good carbs are unrefined, minimally processed carbs that still contain their natural nutrition. Whole grains top the list. These grains are higher in protein, fiber, vitamins, and minerals than their refined counterparts—and you get the net carb advantage when you eat them. For example, semolina-based pasta is out, but whole-wheat pasta is in. White bread is out; various kinds of whole-grain breads are in. Whole grains such as barley, bulgur, wheat berries, wild rice, and brown rice are acceptable. Beans are also in, again in carefully controlled amounts. Beans are nutritional powerhouses with a lot of protein and fiber, but the net carbs can add up fast. The net carbs for different beans vary, so check the tables in this book to find the counts for your favorites.

As you gradually increase your daily net carbs you can also add in some starchier vegetables, such as peas, sweet potatoes, and even white potatoes. Again, the net carbs can add up fast, so check the tables and be aware of portion size.

You can even add fruit back into your diet! Low-carb fruits such as berries are the best choice, but you can really have just about any fresh fruit, as long as you keep an eye on your total net carbs for the day and keep the portion small if necessary. Avoid fruit that has added sugar—fruit cocktail in heavy syrup, for instance.

GOOD FATS, BAD FATS

If you've ever tried to lose weight on the standard low-fat, reduced-calorie diet, you know it was a constant struggle. You felt hungry all the time, even if you'd just eaten a full meal. Not only that, your meals were boring—you got really tired of all those skimpy portions of steamed vegetables and skinless baked chicken. A major reason low-fat diets are so hard to stick with is that dietary fat is what gives a lot of foods their flavor. Dietary fat also plays an important role in satiety—making you feel full and satisfied by your food. And the right kind of dietary fat is actually good for you.

Because one gram of fat has 9 calories, while a gram of carbohydrate or protein has only 4 calories, cutting fat would seem to be a good way to cut back on calories, which in turn would seem to be a good way to lose weight. In addition, saturated fat in the diet—the kind found in meat and dairy products—is often blamed as a factor in causing heart disease from clogged arteries. A low-fat diet would seem to be healthier for your heart as well.

Not so fast. First, cutting back on dietary fat in theory does reduce the number of calories you eat, but the foods you eat won't be as satisfying. A 1-cup serving of plain steamed broccoli seasoned with lemon juice is likely to leave you wanting something a lot more interesting, to say nothing of more satiating. But a cup of broccoli sautéed in olive oil and sprinkled with Parmesan cheese is a lot more enjoyable—and you'll feel full after eating it. Chances are that an hour after a meal containing the steamed broccoli, you'll be hungry again. Unless your willpower is strong that day and every day, you'll soon find yourself snacking on a high-carb, high-calorie food and not losing weight. But when your meal includes the sautéed broccoli with cheese, the olive oil helps your feeling of satiety kick in quickly. Your meal leaves you feeling full, and you stay that way longer.

Your meal is also healthier. Despite all the low-fat hype you hear, fat isn't a deadly substance, and eating it doesn't automatically clog up the arteries of your heart.

Dietary fat falls into three general categories: saturated,

partially unsaturated, and monounsaturated. Many researchers believe that saturated fat, the kind found primarily in animal foods such as beef and dairy products, plays a role in causing heart disease. There's probably some truth to this—particularly if your diet is also high in poor-quality carbohydrates, low in fresh vegetables, and low in the other dietary fats. Many low-carb researchers believe, however, that moderate amounts of saturated fat as part of a balanced low-carbohydrate diet probably don't add to your risk of heart disease. They point out that losing weight, eating more vegetables, and getting more exercise are powerful tools for helping to prevent heart disease—and that's exactly what following the low-carb approach provides.

But what about all the cholesterol that's in animal foods such as meat and eggs? While it's true that these foods contain cholesterol, and that having high low-density lipoprotein cholesterol (LDL or "bad" cholesterol) is undesirable, the cholesterol in your diet doesn't necessarily have a lot to do with the cholesterol in your bloodstream. Your body needs cholesterol—among other things, you use it to make hormones such as testosterone and estrogen, to make walls for the trillions of cells in your body, and to make the fatty sheaths that coat your nerves. You manufacture most of the cholesterol you need in your liver—in most people, well under half of the cholesterol they eat is absorbed. And most people who try to lower their cholesterol levels through the standard low-fat, high-carb diet don't succeed and end up taking expensive statin drugs instead. When they try a low-carb diet, however, they often have remarkable success, even though they don't limit their fat intake. The reasons are complex and not fully understood, but in a number of recent serious studies, dieters who followed a low-carb approach actually lowered their cholesterol more than dieters who followed the low-fat approach (for a list of recent studies, see pages 39–42).

Partially unsaturated fats are found in many plant foods—vegetable oils such as corn oil and canola oil are good examples. Green leafy vegetables and whole grains also contain partially unsaturated fats. The best source, however, is fish. The fat in fish is mostly in the form called omega-3 fatty acids, which have been shown to help prevent heart disease. That's why low-carb diet plans generally call for you to eat fish at least twice a week.

Monounsaturated fats are found in nuts and nut oils, olive oil, and some plant foods such as avocados. The monounsaturated fats may be the healthiest of all. People who follow a traditional Mediterranean diet, for example, often get about 40 percent of their daily calories from fat. That's far above the 30 percent of calories from fat recommended by authorities such as the American Heart Association, yet these people tend to lead long, healthy lives. Why? Because that fat comes mostly from olive oil, with smaller amounts coming from fish, dairy products, whole grains, nuts, and vegetables.

When you start taking the low-carb approach, in many ways you're doing just what those long-living Mediterranean folks do: You're now eating high-quality protein, high-quality dietary fat, unprocessed carbohydrates, and plenty of fresh vegetables, along with some fresh fruit. What aren't you eating? Processed and refined foods, junk food, snack food, sugary food—all the foods that are high in carbohydrates and low in nutrition.

There's one fat that should be avoided at all costs: Trans fats, also called hydrogenated or partially hydrogenated vegetable oil. This is the fat that's used in most baked goods such as cookies, snack cakes, doughnuts, and bread; it's also the fat that's used to produce fried foods in fast food restaurants and packaged foods, and it's the fat that's used in a lot of salty snack foods such as potato chips. Trans fats are made by taking polyunsaturated vegetable oil and processing it until it becomes more saturated. Trans fats have been linked to an increased risk of heart disease, among other health problems. The federal nutritional guidelines now recommend avoiding trans fats as much as possible. If you're still eating high-carb snack foods and fast-food meals, that could be hard to do. If you're following the low-carb approach, however, it's easy, because you're not eating most of the foods that are likely to contain them.

THE EXERCISE CONNECTION

Cutting carbs will almost certainly lead to weight loss if you're overweight, but that's only half the equation. The other half is exercise. To get the most from the low-carb approach, you need to become more physically active as well. In fact, exercise is one of the secrets for low-carb success. The fitter you are, the more muscles you have. And because muscles are more metabolically active than fat, you burn more calories even if you're sitting still. Even better, the more physically active you are, the more you can add in a few more daily carbs and continue to lose weight. Once you've reached your goal weight, staying active helps you stay there and lets you enjoy a somewhat higher daily carb intake.

The exercise program recommended most by doctors is simple: Take a 30-minute walk every day. No expensive gym, no fancy gear, little chance of injury, and no learning curve. Just put on a comfortable pair of shoes and go. Especially when you first start a daily walking program, you don't have to go far or fast. It's the length of your walk, not how much ground you cover, that counts. As you lose weight and get fitter, you can pick up the pace, walk longer, or both.

TWO

Understanding Net Carbs

Net carbs, impact carbs, effective carbs—call them what you want, these carbs are the key to successful low-carb dieting. Let's take a closer look at what they are.

The net carbs in a food are the total carbohydrates in the portion *minus* the fiber. For example, a medium-sized apple has 21 grams of carbohydrates, and it also has 4 grams of fiber. Subtract 4 from 21 and you get 17, the net carbs in an apple. The net carbs are the carbs that will have an effect or an impact on your body—they're the carbs you count.

Why do you subtract the fiber carbs from the total carbs? Because fiber consists of the indigestible parts of plant foods, mostly the cellulose that makes up the cell walls, along with other forms of fiber such as pectin. Technically speaking, fiber is a carbohydrate, but it's so complex that your body doesn't really break it down and digest it—fiber travels through your digestive system pretty much untouched. That means the total amount of carbohydrates in a food according to the food facts label isn't necessarily the amount you absorb. Generally speaking, the more natural and unprocessed a carb-containing food is, the more fiber it will contain as well. (The exception would be dairy foods such as cheese and milk, which have carbs but don't have any fiber.) Start processing the food, however, and most of the fiber disappears. A cup of cooked whole-wheat spaghetti, for instance, has about 37 carb grams and 6 fiber grams, for a net carbs count of 31 grams. A cup of cooked regular spaghetti has nearly 40 carb grams and only about 2 fiber grams, for a net carb count of 38.

What does that tell you? That a diet rich in fresh vegetables, fruits, and whole grains will tend to be a diet that's lower in net carbs. That's one of the reasons a low-carb diet can be so good for your health. The other is that all those veggies, fruits, and grain are also rich in vitamins, minerals, and phytonutrients—all the many natural substances that give these foods their characteristic color and taste. Spinach, for instance, is rich in iron and potassium. It's an excellent source of the crucial B vitamin folate (folic acid), and it's also high in lutein and zeaxanthin, two phytonutrients that help protect your eyes from the sight-robbing disease, age-related macular degeneration. The bonus is that a cup of cooked spinach has nearly 7 grams of carbs and 4 grams of fiber, for a net carb count of only 3 grams.

Sugar alcohols such as maltitol, lactitol, sorbitol are used to sweeten some reduced-carb products. Glycerin and glycerol are also used as sweeteners in these products. Strictly speaking, they're not sugar alcohols, but for carb-counting purposes, they are. The good thing about sugar alcohols is that they get deducted from the total carb count. The reasoning here is that while sugar alcohols are natural sugars, they're much more complex than sucrose, glucose, fructose, and other simple sugars. Like fiber, sugar alcohols are carbohydrates that are so complex that your digestive system can't break them down. They give foods a sweet taste, but like fiber they pass through your body largely undigested. To find the net carbs of a food containing sugar alcohol, simply subtract the sugar alcohol carbs (and any fiber carbs) in the portion from the total carbs. For example, a reduced-carb energy bar that has 21 carb grams might also have 7 fiber grams and 12 sugar alcohol grams, leaving a net carb count of just 2 grams.

When it comes to sugar alcohols, though, you need to be on the cautious side. Some people can get digestive upsets from eating them, and there's some controversy as to exactly how much of the sugar alcohol you really do absorb. And an important part of low-carb dieting is breaking the sweet tooth that helped get you overweight to begin with. Remember that low-carb energy bars, candy, and other sweetened products are meant to be eaten only occasionally.

THE LOW-CARB SECRET

When you count net carbs instead of total carbs, you've learned the true secret of low-carb dieting: By including plenty of foods that have low net carb counts in your diet, you get to eat satisfying portions of a very healthful and varied diet. If you're at or near your goal weight and can raise your carb count, you can now add in more fruit, starchier vegetables, and small portions of high-quality grains and beans and still stay within a daily net carb range that's good for you. Net carbs make dieting easy and hunger-free—and your meals will never be dull.

TRACKING YOUR NET CARBS

Even net carbs can add up, however, especially if you really need to watch your intake. Don't guess when it comes to net carbs. Check out the net carbs of your favorite foods by using this tables in this book. The carb counts, fiber and sugar alcohol (where appropriate) grams, and net carb counts are given for over 2,700 foods.

When you're in the more restrictive phases of a low-carb diet, you may find it easier to write down your daily carb intake. This helps you keep track of the net carb grams and helps you figure out where any excess carbs are coming from. When you've been low-carbing for a while, you'll have a better idea of how to control your carbs and may not need to watch the net carb grams as closely. If your weight loss stalls or you start gaining, however, start tracking those net carbs carefully again. Chances are you've let too many carbs creep back into your diet. Hunt those carbs down and eliminate them, and your weight loss is likely to resume.

NET CARBS AND THE FOOD LABEL

Because low-carbing has become such a popular approach to weight loss and better health, today many food manufacturers are making products designed to help low-carb dieters. These products can be very, very helpful. Low-carb energy bars, for instance, make a good meal substitute, and low-carb candy is useful for those times when you simply have to have some chocolate. Low-carb versions of pasta, milk, and other basic foods are also convenient and tasty.

To lower the carbs in a food, manufacturers use a variety of techniques. In baked goods, soy flour can be substituted for wheat flour, or extra fiber such as oat bran can be added. For sweetened products such as low-carb candy, sugar alcohols such as maltitol, lactitol, or sorbitol are used. Sometimes the manufacturer simply makes the portion smaller so it will contain fewer carbs.

There's a problem with low-carb foods, however. Nobody can define exactly what they are. When a manufacturer says on the packaging that a food is low fat, for instance, that claim is regulated by the federal Food and Drug Administration (FDA) and has a very specific meaning. Ditto for any other food label claims that use the words "low," "reduced," or "free." Although the FDA has defined the meanings of these terms for many nutrients such as salt and fat, it hasn't done so yet for carbohydrates (though they're working on it). That means food manufacturers can't use phrases like "low-carb," "reduced-carb," "carb-free," or "only 2 carbs" on their labels. Instead, they work around the issue by giving the total net carbs for the food, or using phrases such as "carb smart" or "carb aware."

What does this mean for the consumer? Caution, as always. For high-carb foods, even cutting the carb count in half could still leave the food higher in carbs than you want. A manufacturer could label a product "carb smart" and say it has only 1 carb per portion, but if the portion size for 1 carb is very small, you might easily eat several portions and end up getting more carbs than you realize—and even small portions of low-carb foods add up. Evaluate the claims on other food packages carefully as well. A food that claims to be "fat free" or to have "no added sugars" could still be high in carbs. And don't forget that high-calorie foods tend to also be high-carbohydrate foods.

To be sure you're not going overboard with carbs, use the tables in this book. Where possible, also look at the packaging and read the food facts label carefully. Check the portion size and eyeball it against the package size to get an idea of how large the portion really is. Check the carbohydrate count and then subtract any fiber or sugar alcohols to get the net carbs per portion.

Convenient as low-carb foods can be, save them for occasional use. They're no substitute for the fresh vegetables, whole grains, and high-quality protein that a low-carb diet emphasizes.

FINDING HIDDEN CARBS

Packaged foods can be a major pitfall for low-carb dieters—these foods often contain hidden carbs. To find them, read the packaging carefully. Watch out for packaging that says "no sugar added" or "contains only natural sugars." These products may still be high in carbs, even if they don't have any added sugar. Read the serving size carefully too. A single serving of the food might not have many carbs, but the serving could be so small that you'll end up eating a lot more than you realize.

Another way to hide the carbs is to disguise the sugar under another name. Check the ingredients list. If it contains any of these words, be wary:

- brown sugar
- corn sweetener
- corn syrup
- dextrose
- fructose
- fruit juice concentrate
- galactose
- glucose
- high-fructose corn syrup
- honey
- invert sugar
- lactose
- levulose
- maltose
- malt

- malt syrup
- maple sugar
- maple syrup
- molasses
- raw sugar
- sucrose (table sugar)

To reduce the carb count in sweet foods such as candy, manufacturers use sugar alcohols such as maltitol or artificial sweeteners such as sucralose (Splenda®), aspartame (NutraSweet®) and saccharin (Sweet 'N Low®). Products made with artificial sweeteners are acceptable on low-carb diets. They're fine for home use as well. Sucralose can even be used in baking.

LOW-CARBING AND THE GLYCEMIC INDEX

In recent years the glycemic index (GI) has become a very useful addition to the low-carb approach. That's because the glycemic index is a good way to judge both the quantity and quality of the carbohydrates in a food. Here's how it works:

As you understand by now, refined carbohydrates have a very rapid impact on your blood sugar, because they are digested quickly and are absorbed quickly. Unrefined carbohydrates and carbohydrate-containing foods that are high in fiber are digested more slowly and absorbed into your bloodstream slowly and steadily. They have a much lower impact on your blood sugar. The glycemic index is a way of measuring exactly how much of an effect a particular food actually has on your blood sugar. To find the glycemic index of a particular food, volunteers eat it on an empty stomach and then have their blood sugar measured at intervals over the next few hours. The results are compared to the effect of table sugar (sucrose) on your blood sugar. Because the glucose from table sugar hits your bloodstream almost at once, it's rated at 100 on the glycemic index. All other foods are compared to that number. The lower the glycemic index number, then, the less of an impact that particular food has on your blood sugar.

In general, any food with a glycemic index number under 55 is considered low. If the GI of the food is between 56 and 69, it's an intermediate GI food; above 70, it's a high GI food. Overall, foods that are low in carbohydrates and high in fiber are low-GI foods that will have a lower impact on your blood sugar. A pear, for instance, has about 11 net carbs and a GI of 38. A baked potato has 30 net carbs and a GI of 85.

The glycemic index was developed as a way to help people with diabetes select foods that would have the least impact on their blood sugar. It's not primarily designed as a way to lose weight. If you select low-GI foods, you're also usually selecting foods that are lower in carbohydrates, but some foods that are fairly high in carbs are relatively low on the glycemic index. For example, 1 cup of cooked barley has 42 net carbs, but a GI of only 25. If you're in the weight-loss phase of a low-carb diet, this would still be a food to avoid.

Researchers have taken the glycemic index concept a step further with the idea of the glycemic load. This is a way to look at both the carbohydrates and the fiber in a standard portion of a food and assess the impact on blood sugar. It's a little more complicated than the glycemic index, but it gives you a better idea of which foods to select. Let's look at an example: One medium apple has a GI value of 40 and has 15 grams of carbohydrate. To calculate the glycemic load, multiply 40 by 15 and divide by 100 to get 6 (40 x 15 ÷ 100 = 6). Compare that to the glycemic load for 8 ounces of unsweetened apple juice. The GI of the juice is also 40, but because it has a lot less fiber, you absorb a lot more carbohydrate when you drink it—29 grams in all. When you work out the numbers, the glycemic load of the juice is 12, or double the impact of eating an apple. Clearly, if you need to keep an eye on your blood sugar, the apple is the better choice.

Fortunately, you don't have to work out the glycemic load numbers for most commonly eaten foods. You can easily look them up in the standard work on the subject, *The New Glucose Revolution* by Jennie Brand-Miller and her colleagues (Marlowe, 1999), and in related books. Even if you don't have GI and GL tables handy, a good rule of thumb is that the more fiber and fewer carbs a food has, the lower the GI and GL numbers will be. Another good rule of thumb is that most foods with a GI below 55 are acceptable on a low-carb diet.

THREE

Low-Carb Living

Choosing to follow the low-carb approach isn't going on a diet—it's making a lifestyle decision. It's surprisingly easy to stick with your low-carb choice, because the foods you eat are basically the same foods that everyone else eats—minus the low-quality, nutritionally poor carbs. Even so, you need to be aware of the danger areas that can allow unwanted carbohydrates to creep back into your diet.

PORTION SIZE PITFALLS

Here's a typical dinner for someone on a low-carb diet:

- large green salad with vinaigrette or blue cheese dressing
- grilled chicken breast
- broccoli sautéed in olive oil with slivered almonds
- strawberries with real whipped cream (artificially sweetened)

Total carbs for this satisfying, tasty, and very healthy

meal: about 15. Meals like this make low-carbing very easy to live with in the long run.

You may have noticed that this meal isn't measured out into portions based on calories and fat grams. A big reason so many people achieve success with low-carb dieting is that they don't have to measure out portions, count calories, or ever go hungry. Instead, you choose foods that are low in net carbs, always have protein and dietary fat along with your carbs, and eat portions that satisfy you. Another great beauty of the low-carb approach is that your food really does satisfy you—and quickly. Because you eat plenty of fresh vegetables and high-quality protein and don't have to skimp on dietary fat, you fill up *fast*. This is part of the reason low-carb dieting works: Because your food is so satisfying and because you don't get hungry again so soon after eating it, you tend to take in fewer calories.

But even on a low-carb diet, you need to be aware of two pitfalls: portion size and overeating.

Portion size is key, because it's all too easy to underestimate the size of your portion and therefore the net carbs it contains. Today the standard portion size of many prepared and restaurant foods is very large—often much larger than the standard sizes nutritionists use when they give nutrient counts in books like this. When your portions are larger than you realize, you end up with more carbs—sometimes a lot more carbs—than you realize. That can lead to stalled weight loss, which in turn leads you to get frustrated and abandon your diet.

To avoid going that route, learn to estimate your portion sizes accurately. It's easy to do—half an hour in the kitchen is all it takes.

Using a standard measuring cup, measure out a 1-cup portion of salad greens. Do the same for a ½-cup portion of cooked vegetables and pasta or rice. Take a good look at the portions while they're still in the measuring cup, and then put them onto a standard dinner plate and look them over again. You'll quickly get a good idea of what a cup of salad greens looks like. You'll probably also realize that half a cup of cooked rice or pasta is a lot less than you thought. Once you have a better grasp of portion size, you'll find it easier to estimate your carb intake correctly.

The standard portion of many foods is by weight, not volume. By using a kitchen scale or a postage scale, you can get a handle on these portions too. For example, to get a good idea of how many nuts are in an ounce, weigh some out. You might be surprised to realize that an ounce of almonds is about 22 nuts. That's a lot of almonds—a great snack that has only 2 net carbs and 10 grams of healthy monounsaturated fat. An ounce of cheese is another important measurement for low-carb dieters. Weigh out some slices of your favorite cheese to get an idea of how it looks.

Of course, you can't carry a measuring cup and kitchen scale with you everywhere, so you need another way to estimate portions when you're away from home. Here are some good ways to visualize portion size:

- 3-ounce bagel = 1 can tuna
- ½ cup cooked rice or pasta = the amount that would fill half a tennis ball
- 3 ounces beef, pork, chicken, fish = a deck of cards
- 1 ounce of cheese = a pair of dice
- 1 cup salad greens = the size of your fist
- 1 ounce nuts = a handful
- 1 cup cooked vegetables = a tennis ball

Once you have a good handle on your portion sizes, it's time to tackle the overeating question. Following a low-carb diet means not being overly concerned about portions of low-carb foods. It *doesn't* mean, however, that you can overeat. When you have a meal, go for portions that leave you satisfied—not stuffed. You can still eat large portions of salad and low-carb vegetables, and you don't have to measure out your protein and fat portions. The combination of vegetables, protein, and fat at a meal should fill you up quickly, but many of us have a tendency to keep eating after we're full. We don't always hear the signals our body sends to tell us we've had enough.

There are some tried-and-true tricks for learning to control your appetite:

- Don't get too hungry for your main meals—when you're ravenous you're more likely to choose foods that aren't the best for you. You're also much more likely to overeat. If you get hungry between meals, don't resist. Instead, have a snack that includes some protein and fat—a celery stick stuffed with cream cheese, for example.
- Begin your meal with a cup of hot soup—it will help fill you up without adding a lot of carbs. Ditto for a large salad.
- After you've eaten your meal, you may still feel hungry even though you've had satisfying portions. Why? Your brain hasn't caught up with your stomach yet and is still sending you hunger signals. Be aware of this possibility and wait 10 minutes or longer before going back for seconds. At that point you'll probably find you're not hungry any more.
- Still want those seconds? Have them—but not just of your favorite food. Include small portions of each food in the meal on your seconds plate.
- After finishing your meal, wait 10 to 20 minutes before having dessert. That gives your body a chance

to stop sending hunger signals and diminishes your appetite for dessert.

- If you do want dessert, make a good, low-carb choice such as fresh berries, sugar-free gelatin, or low-carb ice cream.
- Skimping on the carbs during the meal so you can splurge on dessert isn't a good idea. You'll have a hard time sticking to a small portion. Even worse, eating a rich dessert may trigger your sweet tooth and derail your low-carb approach.

If you consistently find yourself overeating, ask yourself why. Are you truly hungry, or are you just bored? Or maybe you're angry? Stressed? Depressed? Are you rewarding yourself with food? Is eating just a habit, something you do automatically in front of the TV? Be honest with yourself and you may be able to get a better understanding of how your emotions and your appetite are connected.

If you catch yourself eating for reasons other than genuine hunger, try doing something else instead. Call a friend, go for a walk, do your exercise routine, take up knitting or another activity that keeps your hands busy—even do housework! And if the urge to eat is irresistible, choose a low-carb food. Cucumber spears and blue cheese dip are a much better choice than potato chips.

LOW-CARB SWITCHEROOS

Trading in high-carb foods for lower-carb alternatives is surprisingly easy. Simply selecting from the many sugar-free products that have been on the grocery shelves for years can cut a lot of carbs. Look for sugar-free pudding, gelatin desserts, hot chocolate, candy, iced tea, soda, and other foods. But read the labels carefully—products such as sugar-free cookies can still be high in carbs. Today there are also plenty of reduced-carb products to choose from for common foods such as breakfast cereal, bread, shakes, and even pasta. You can almost always find at least some of these products in the grocery store. But you don't have to buy a lot of special foods to make low-carbing a regular part of your life. You can easily make a lot of simple low-carb switches just by substituting one standard food for another. Here's how:

High-carb food	Low-carb alternative
banana	apple or pear
breakfast cereal	oatmeal or no-sugar-added granola
cottage cheese	cream cheese
crackers	celery sticks, baby carrots, bell pepper strips
croutons	slivered almonds
flour tortilla	corn tortilla
french toast	scrambled eggs
mashed potatoes	mashed turnips or cauliflower
potato chips	dry-roasted nuts
potato salad	cole slaw
pretzels	air-popped popcorn
soda pop	diet soda, club soda, mineral water
spaghetti	spaghetti squash
sugar	sucralose or other artificial sweetener
white bread	100% whole-wheat bread
yogurt with sweetened fruit	plain yogurt with berries or fresh fruit

A little imagination and you'll easily discover your own low-carb alternatives.

EATING OUT THE LOW-CARB WAY

So many people are now eating the low-carb way that restaurants have very quickly learned to accommodate them. Many restaurants now have special low-carb items on the menu, but at any restaurant today, it's perfectly acceptable to ask for broccoli instead of mashed potatoes, or to ask for a half-size portion of pasta. Even so, eating out can test your ability to stick to your low-carb decisions, especially when the dessert menu comes along. Try these tips for keeping the carbs down:

- Have a salad as your appetizer—but watch out for the high-carb add-ons like croutons. Also, salad dressings can contain added sugar. Blue cheese, ranch, and vinaigrette dressings are the safest bets.
- Ask to substitute vegetables for pasta, rice, potatoes, and other high-carb side dishes.
- Avoid deep-fried, breaded, or battered foods.
- Ask your server to take the bread basket away—or at least keep it on the opposite side of the table from you.
- You don't have to clean your plate—if the portion is large, eat only enough to satisfy your appetite and ask for a doggy bag for the rest.
- It's OK to eat dessert if you're having a festive or celebratory meal—a birthday dinner, for instance. Plan ahead by cutting back a bit on your carbs for a few days beforehand, and keep the carbs down by asking for a half-size portion or sharing the dessert

with someone. And remember, you don't have to eat it all.

Some cuisines are better choices than others for low-carb dieting. It's hard to avoid carbs at a pizza restaurant, for example, and most fast-food restaurants will have only a limited selection of low-carb choices. By choosing carefully, however, and asking for low-carb substitutions whenever possible, it's easy to enjoy just about any kind of restaurant.

SUPPLEMENTS AND LOW-CARB DIETING

Do you need extra vitamins and minerals from supplements while you're on a low-carb diet? It's hard to say with any certainty. On the one hand, because you're now eating so many fresh fruits, vegetables, and whole grains, you're probably getting more of these important natural substances from your food than ever before. On the other hand, most of us can't manage to eat well every single day, so just about all nutrition experts suggest that everyone take a good multivitamin with minerals every day—it's a very inexpensive way to make sure you're getting daily minimums. But do you need the special supplements formulated just for low-carb dieters? The primary additional element in these supplements is extra B vitamins. That's because in the standard American diet, most people get a lot of their daily Bs, especially folic acid, from the vitamins that are added back into enriched white flour. So, the thinking goes, if you're no longer eating foods made with enriched white flour, you're not getting enough B vitamins. But in reality, low-carb dieters get plenty of all the B vitamins, because these vitamins are found in abundance in nuts, beans, meat, milk, whole grains, eggs, and dark-green leafy vegetables, among other foods. You're very unlikely to be deficient in B vitamins if you cut out refined grain foods from your diet. One exception might be women of child-bearing age, who should get at least 400 micrograms of folic acid daily to help prevent birth defects. If you fall into this category, discuss your dietary supplements with your doctor.

Supplements called starch blockers are marketed to dieters as a way to eat carbs but keep them from being absorbed by your body. These products contain amylase inhibitors, which are made from a protein found in white kidney beans *(Phaseolus vulgaris)*. The idea is that the amylase inhibitor keeps starch molecules from being broken down by digestive juices in your stomach and absorbed into your bloodstream. In theory, the starch has been "neutralized" and will then pass through and out of your digestive tract without any further absorption. There are some problems with the theory, though. The research the manufacturers use to tout their products comes from a supplement company that makes a starch blocker. It's not objective or reliable. The manufacturers claim that you lose weight by taking their starch blockers, and they say amylase inhibitors works much like the prescription drug acarbose (Precose™). The problem is that no study of acarbose has ever shown that it helps people lose weight—it's used primarily to help people control their blood sugar. More seriously, the manufacturers of starch blockers conveniently forget to mention that when undigested carbohydrates enter your intestines, they *do* get digested further, by the natural bacteria there. The result is fermentation. In other words, gas—and lots of it, sometimes accompanied by severe diarrhea. There are some people whose digestive systems aren't affected by starch blockers, but the only way you'll know you're one of them is to try it. Why take the risk? Staying away from the carbs to begin with is a better approach.

CARB CRAVINGS

Carb cravings can be a problem for some people, especially when they first start low-carbing and are in the most restrictive phase. When you're in the throes of a carb craving attack, you'll eat just about anything that's sweet or starchy. Cravings can be caused by a lot of things: stress, anxiety, depression, tension, anger, boredom, tiredness, or just feeling a need for the emotional comfort food can bring. You probably won't be able to stop a craving with simple willpower—the feeling is too intense for that. Instead, try some techniques that incorporate low-carb principles:

- Often cravings happen because your blood sugar is low. Keep up your blood sugar and you may be able to stop cravings before they start. Try eating a small meal or snack that contains some protein and dietary fat every few hours. Examples: hard-boiled egg, string cheese, celery stick stuffed with cream cheese or peanut butter.
- If you must have something sweet, try a piece of fresh fruit. Have some protein and fat with it—a piece of cheese or some nuts, for example.
- If you're really craving something starchy, try a whole-wheat pita or other whole-grain food—and have some protein and dietary fat with it.
- Gotta have chocolate? Choose a sugar-free brand.
- Be careful about alcohol—it can trigger cravings.
- Are you getting enough sleep? You're less likely to crave the energy lift of high-carb foods if you're well rested.

Sometimes you just can't fight off a carb attack. When it happens, don't beat yourself up or decide that you can't stick to a low-carb diet. Think about what caused the attack, try to find ways to avoid that situation in the future or deal with it more constructively, and get right back on the low-carb track.

HOLIDAYS AND SPECIAL OCCASIONS

Your low-carb diet doesn't have to go out the window when holidays and special occasions arrive. Traditionally these events mean high-carb treats like pies, cakes, and cookies, but they also include lower-carb foods such as roast turkey, ham, and vegetables. Enjoy small portions of the special foods you get only around a particular holiday—Thanksgiving wouldn't be Thanksgiving without pumpkin pie—and make the best choices you can among the other lower-carb foods. Similarly, when you're celebrating a special event, enjoy a small amount of high-carb food as part of the fun. Stay aware that this is a special occasion, though, and that the foods you're eating are special too. The next day, get firmly back into the low-carb groove. After you've been low-carbing for a while, you'll probably find that it's much easier to stick to small tastes of the high-carb foods. Many people find that after a few months of the low-carb approach, rich desserts taste almost unbearably sweet and that they can eat only small portions.

FOUR

Low-Carb Diets and Your Health

Today nearly two-thirds of all adult Americans are over-weight; 30 percent are obese. That means two out of three adults have an increased risk of diabetes, high blood pressure, heart disease, cancer, stroke, and arthritis.

If you're carrying around too many extra pounds, chances are you know it already. What you may not know is exactly how much heavier you are than would be best for you. Fortunately, there's an easy and accurate way to find where you stand. It's called the Body Mass Index, or BMI for short. The BMI uses the ratio of your height to your weight to tell you if you're overweight, and if so, by how much. One advantage of the BMI is that it presents your weight in a range, not a single number. The BMI ranges take into account things like having a slight or heavy build. The BMI lets you see easily where your current weight is relative to a healthier weight range for you. Use the BMI table on page 32 to find your current weight, determine if you're overweight or obese and by how much, and find the healthier weight range for your height.

Body Mass Index (BMI) Table

BMI	19	20	21	22	23	24	25	26	27	28	29	30	31	32	33	34	35	36	37	38	39	40
Height (inches)									Body Weight (pounds)													
58	91	96	100	105	110	115	119	124	129	134	138	143	148	153	158	162	167	172	177	181	186	191
59	94	99	104	109	114	119	124	128	133	138	143	148	153	158	163	168	173	178	183	188	193	198
60	97	102	107	112	118	123	128	133	138	143	148	153	158	163	168	174	179	184	189	194	199	204
61	100	106	111	116	122	127	132	137	143	148	153	158	164	169	174	180	185	190	195	201	206	211
62	104	109	115	120	126	131	136	142	147	153	158	164	169	175	180	186	191	196	202	207	213	218
63	107	113	118	124	130	135	141	146	152	158	163	169	175	180	186	191	197	203	208	214	220	225
64	110	116	122	128	134	140	145	151	157	163	169	174	180	186	192	197	204	209	215	221	227	232
65	114	120	126	132	138	144	150	156	162	168	174	180	186	192	198	204	210	216	222	228	234	240
66	118	124	130	136	142	148	155	161	167	173	179	186	192	198	204	210	216	223	229	235	241	247
67	121	127	134	140	146	153	159	166	172	178	185	191	198	204	211	217	223	230	236	242	249	255
68	125	131	138	144	151	158	164	171	177	184	190	197	203	210	216	223	230	236	243	249	256	262
69	128	135	142	149	155	162	169	176	182	189	196	203	209	216	223	230	236	243	250	257	263	270
70	132	139	146	153	160	167	174	181	188	195	202	209	216	222	229	236	243	250	257	264	271	278
71	136	143	150	157	165	172	179	186	193	200	208	215	222	229	236	243	250	257	265	272	279	286
72	140	147	154	162	169	177	184	191	199	206	213	221	228	235	242	250	258	265	272	279	287	294
73	144	151	159	166	174	182	189	197	204	212	219	227	235	242	250	257	265	272	280	288	295	302
74	148	155	163	171	179	186	194	202	210	218	225	233	241	249	256	264	272	280	287	295	303	311
75	152	160	168	176	184	192	200	208	216	224	232	240	248	256	264	272	279	287	295	303	311	319
76	156	164	172	180	189	197	205	213	221	230	238	246	254	263	271	279	287	295	304	312	320	328

Source: National Institutes of Health

To use this chart, find your height in inches in the left-hand column labeled Height, then move across to find your weight (in pounds). The number at the top of that column is the BMI at that height and weight.

BMI between 20 and 24.9: normal weight for your height
BMI between 25 and 29.9: overweight
BMI 30 and up: obese
BMI over 40: severely obese

Another way to look at your weight is to look at your waist measurement. If you're a woman with a waist measurement of more than 35 inches or a man with a waist measurement of more than 40 inches, you're overweight or obese.

No matter how you look at it, the higher up you move on the BMI table or the bigger your waist measurement is, the more those extra pounds are a risk to your health. In addition to an increased risk of severe health problems such as high blood pressure, diabetes, and certain types of cancer, your chances of dying prematurely go up as your weight does. Compared to people who are in the normal BMI range, obese people (BMI of 30 or more) have a 50 to 100 percent increased risk of death from all causes.

Sadly, many people who are overweight have tried diet after diet. They've lost weight, only to gain it back and then some as soon as they went off whatever restrictive diet they were on. It's a cycle that leaves them heavier, unhealthier, and unhappier each time.

For many, the low-carb approach has been the way out of diet despair. Low-carbing works because it's not a diet—it's a lifestyle. You don't eat special foods, drink special shakes, or go to meetings. You don't weigh out portions, count calories or fat grams, or worry over every mouthful. And best of all, you don't go hungry.

What do you do? You simply substitute healthy, delicious, low-carb choices for the high-carb, low-nutrition foods that are the true culprits in today's obesity epidemic. It's a sensible approach, one that's easy to make part of your lifestyle and stay with for a lifetime.

IS LOW-CARBING SAFE?

You've probably heard all sorts of warnings about how unhealthy a low-carb diet is. You've been told that ketosis can damage your kidneys and that the diet will thin your bones and clog your arteries. You've also been told that the weight loss is just "water weight" and that you'll gain it all back as soon as you go off the diet.

At this point low-carbohydrate diets have been carefully studied for a long time (see the research papers listed at the end of this chapter). Time after time, low-carb dieting has been shown to be safe for most people.

Let's look at the ketosis question first, because that's the biggest misconception of all about low-carb dieting. When your body starts to use fat for fuel instead of glucose, it does so by breaking the fat down into ketones, chemicals your cells can burn for energy. When weight loss is rapid, you produce more ketones than you can use. To get rid of them, your body excretes them in your breath and in your urine. If you're excreting a lot of extra ketones, you're in ketosis. There's nothing dangerous about ketosis—in fact, many people are in mild ketosis when they wake up in the morning after not eating for a number of hours. The misconception about ketosis comes from confusing it with ketoacidosis, a dangerous condition with a similar-sounding name.

Ketoacidosis can occur in people with Type 1 diabetes, where the pancreas no longer produces insulin, the hormone that carries glucose into the body's cells to be used as fuel. If you have Type 1 diabetes, you must inject yourself with insulin several times a day. If you don't, your blood sugar can build up to dangerously high levels because it can't get into your cells. Your body will get desperate for energy and start breaking down fat so rapidly that the sudden huge amount of ketones makes your blood too acidic. This very dangerous condition is known as ketoacidosis. If it goes on for long, it can lead to coma and death. Ketoacidosis is a very serious problem for people with Type 1 diabetes, but it is almost impossible for anyone else. Even if you have Type 2 diabetes (also sometimes called adult-onset diabetes), ketoacidosis is very, very unlikely to occur on a low-carb diet.

There's also no evidence that ketosis is dangerous for anyone with normal kidneys. If you have kidney disease, however, ketosis might be harmful, and you may need to limit protein in your diet. Eating a low-carb diet, however, doesn't have to mean eating a lot more protein. In fact, most people following low-carb diets eat about the same amounts of protein that they did before going on the diet. A low-carb diet isn't the same thing as a high-protein diet!

When you go on a low-carb diet, ketosis usually occurs only in the most restrictive phase, when carbs are kept to a minimum. For most people, that phase goes on for just a couple of weeks. Even though ketosis is safe for most people, if you want to avoid it, just skip the earliest stage of your low-carb diet plan and start with the lowest carb level of the second step.

Although some people who go on a low-carb diet do excrete a little more calcium than before for the first few weeks, there's no evidence that the calcium is coming from your bones or thinning them in any way. And as you know from the discussion of dietary fat you just read, eating fat doesn't necessarily make you fat, and it doesn't necessarily raise your blood cholesterol.

What about the water weight? At the start of just about any diet, the first few pounds to come off are often "water weight" from retained fluids caused by the unhealthy diet you were eating before. It's no different on a low-carb diet. But what about after that? The weight you lose after those first few pounds is mostly body fat. As for gaining weight back, that's true of any diet if you go back to your old eating patterns. The low-carb difference is that you can stick to it without feeling hungry, deprived, or bored by your food.

PREDIABETES AND DIABETES

If you're overweight or obese, your chances of having prediabetes or Type 2 diabetes are significantly higher than if you are normal weight. According to the National Institutes of Health, nearly 70 percent of people with Type 2 diabetes have BMIs over 27. (Type 1 diabetes, a much rarer disease, occurs when your pancreas no longer produces insulin. Because at least 90 percent of people with diabetes have Type 2, that's what will be discussed here.) Diabetes is a very serious condition that can lead to a number of dangerous complications, including blindness, kidney failure, and amputations. Someone without diabetes has roughly a 50 percent chance of dying of heart disease. For someone with diabetes, that risk jumps to about 75 percent. And overall, if you have diabetes, your risk of dying is about twice that of someone without diabetes.

Today over 18 million adult Americans have Type 2 diabetes—and the number is growing rapidly. In addition, millions more have prediabetes and will almost certainly develop diabetes if they don't lose weight, exercise more, and change their eating patterns.

Clearly, diabetes is a dangerous disease. Prediabetes can

be almost as bad, because it almost always signals that real diabetes is just around the corner. Let's take a closer look at both conditions and how a low-carb diet can help.

In both prediabetes and diabetes, your body no longer uses blood sugar (glucose) correctly; you have high blood sugar because the glucose is staying in your bloodstream instead of being used in your cells. In both conditions, your blood sugar is high because your cells no longer respond properly to the hormone insulin—the difference between the two conditions is just a matter of degree. Another way to say this is that you have become insulin resistant. Because your cells don't respond well to insulin's signal telling them to let the glucose in to be used as fuel, a lot of it stays in your bloodstream instead. When you first become insulin resistant, your pancreas pours out extra insulin as a way to force your cells to take in glucose. After years of excess production, however, your pancreas wears out and produces less and less insulin. At that point, you may need to inject yourself with insulin several times a day.

The symptoms of prediabetes and diabetes are subtle at first. Because your cells are starved for fuel, you start feeling tired more often. In addition, you may start feeling hungry and thirsty more than before, and you'll probably have to urinate more too. Your blood pressure and blood cholesterol creep up along with your weight. All that extra sugar does a lot of silent damage, especially to the smallest blood vessels in your body. Among other things, high blood sugar can damage your kidneys, your eyes, and the circulation to your feet. High blood sugar is also closely connected to high blood cholesterol and high blood pressure, which in turn means your risk of heart disease skyrockets. Unfortunately, too many people don't learn that they have prediabetes or diabetes until their levels of insulin resistance and blood sugar have become quite high and a lot of damage has already been done. In fact, many don't learn they have diabetes until they're in the emergency room being treated for a heart attack.

If your doctor suspects prediabetes or diabetes, the diagnosis is confirmed by having a blood test. According to the American Diabetes Association, if your fasting blood sugar (taken after not eating for at least 8 hours) is between 100 and 125 milligrams per deciliter (mg/dl), you have impaired fasting glucose (IFG), also known as prediabetes. You have progressed to Type 2 diabetes if your fasting blood sugar is 126 mg/dl or higher, or if your blood sugar two hours after a high-carb meal is 200 mg/dl or higher.

Insulin resistance is almost always caused by a combination of several factors. The first is genetic. If you have a family history of diabetes, you're more likely to get it yourself. There's not much you can do about that, but you can certainly do something about two other factors that play a key role: being overweight or obese and having a sedentary lifestyle.

Losing even a relatively small amount of weight—just 10 percent of your body weight—usually helps insulin resistance quite a bit. So does getting more exercise. Walking for just half an hour a day can make a big difference in insulin resistance.

But for people with prediabetes and diabetes, controlling blood sugar and keeping it as close to normal as possible is just as important as weight loss and exercise. By keeping your blood sugar down, you help minimize the damage to your kidneys, eyes, and other parts of your body, and you help keep your cholesterol and blood pressure down too. Here's where a low-carb diet can be particularly helpful. Put very simply, eating carbohydrates makes your blood sugar go up; cutting back on carbs can help keep your blood sugar down. (There's nowhere near enough space in this book to go into the details—read *Atkins Diabetes Revolution* for an excellent explanation of how low-carbing helps people with blood sugar problems.) By following a low-carb approach, people with prediabetes and diabetes can also often minimize the blood sugar ups and downs that can lead to episodes of hypoglycemia (blood sugar that drops too low).

Low-carb dieting as a treatment for prediabetes and diabetes is controversial. Organizations such as the American Diabetes Association recommend a low-fat diet with as much as 60 percent of calories coming from carbohydrates. The reasoning is that because diabetes sharply raises your blood cholesterol and heart risk, a low-fat diet is the best approach to prevent heart disease. Today, however, more and more doctors are coming to realize that diabetes is a disease of impaired carbohydrate metabolism. They feel it doesn't make sense to have someone with insulin resistance eat a lot of carbohydrates and that a low-carbohydrate diet may be a better approach. How you decide to treat prediabetes or diabetes is an important decision. If you want to try a low-carb diet to help control your blood sugar, discuss your plans with your doctor first.

LOW-CARBOHYDRATE DIET RESEARCH

The scientific evidence for the value of low-carb dieting continues to grow. Some of the most important recent articles in scientific and medical journals are listed below.

Aude, Y. W., Agatson, A.S., Lopez-Jimenez, F., Lieberman, E.H., Almon, M., Hansen, M., Rojas, G., Lamas, G.A., and Hennekens, C.H. "The National Cholesterol Education Program Diet vs a Diet Lower in Carbohydrates and Higher in Protein and Monounsaturated Fat," *Archives of Internal Medicine,* 164, 2004, pp. 2141-2146.

Bode, G., Sargard, K., Homko, C., Mozzoli, M., and Stein, T.P. "Effect of a Low-Carbohydrate Diet on Appetite,

Blood Glucose Levels, and Insulin Resistance in Obese Patients with Type 2 Diabetes," *Annals of the Internal Medicine,* 142(6), 2005, pp. 403-411.

Bravata, D.M., Sanders, L., and Huang, J., et al. "Efficacy and Safety of Low-Carbohydrate Diets: A Systematic Review," *The Journal of the American Medical Association,* 289(14), 2003, pp. 1837-1850.

Brehm, B.J., Spang, S.E., Lattin, B.L., Seeley, R.J., Daniels, S.R., and D'Alessio, D.A. "The Role of Energy Expenditure in the Differential Weight Loss in Obese Women on Low-Fat and Low-Carbohydrate Diets," *Journal of Clinical Endocrinology and Metabolism,* 90(3), 2005, pp. 1475-1482.

Farnsworth, E., Luscombe, N.D., and Noakes, M., et al. "Effect of a High-Protein, Energy-Restricted Diet on Body Composition, Glycemic Control, and Lipid Concentrations in Overweight and Obese Hyperinsulinemic Men and Women," *American Journal of Clinical Nutrition,* 78(1), 2003, pp. 31-39.

Foster, G.D., Wyatt, H.R., and Hill, J.O., et al. "A Randomized Trial of a Low-Carbohydrate Diet for Obesity," *The New England Journal of Medicine,* 348(21), 2003, pp. 2082-2090.

Manninen, A.H. "High-Protein Weight Loss Diets and Purported Adverse Effects: Where is the Evidence," *Sports Nutrition Review Journal,* 2004, 1(1), pp. 45-51.

Meckling, K.A., O'Sullivan, C., and Saari, D. "Comparison of a Low-Fat Diet to a Low-Carbohydrate Diet on Weight Loss, Body Composition, and Risk Factors for Diabetes and Cardiovascular Disease in Free-Living, Overweight Men and Women," *Journal of Clinical Endocrinology and Metabolism,* 89(6), 2004, pp. 2717-2723.

Samaha, F.F., Iqbal, N., and Seshadri, P., et al. "A Low-Carbohydrate as Compared With a Low-Fat Diet in Severe Obesity," *The New England Journal of Medicine,* 348(21), 2003, pp. 2074-2081.

Sharman, M.J., and Volek, J.S. "Weight Loss Leads to Reductions in Inflammatory Biomarkers after a Very Low-Carbohydrate and Low-Fat Diet in Overweight Men," *Clinical Science* (London), 2004.

Stern, L., Iqbal, N., and Seshadri, P., et al. "The Effects of Low-Carbohydrate Versus Conventional Weight Loss Diets in Severely Obese Adults: One-Year Follow-up of a Randomized Trial," *Annals of Internal Medicine,* 140(10), 2004, pp. 778-785.

Volek, J.S., Sharman, M.J., and Gomez A.L., et al. "An Isoenergetic Very Low Carbohydrate Diet Improves Serum HDL Cholesterol and Triacylglycerol Concentrations, the Total Cholesterol to HDL Cholesterol Ratio and Postprandial Lipemic Responses Compared with a Low Fat Diet in Normal Weight, Normolipidemic Women," *The Journal of Nutrition,* 133(9), 2003, pp. 2756-2761.

Volek, J.S., Sharman, M.J., and Gomez, A.L. "Comparison of a Very Low-Carbohydrate and Low-Fat Diet on Fasting Lipids, LDL Subclasses, Insulin Resistance, and Postprandial Lipemic Responses in Overweight Women," *Journal of the American College of Nutrition,* 23(2), 2004, pp. 177-184.

Volek, J.S., and Westman, E.C. "Very-Low-Carbohydrate Weight-Loss Diets Revisited," *Cleveland Clinic Journal of Medicine,* 69(11), 2002, pp. 849-862.

Willett, W.C. "Reduced-Carbohydrate Diets: No Roll in Weight Management?" *Annals of Internal Medicine,* 140(10), 2004, pp. 836-837.

Yancy, W.S., Foy, M.E., and Westman, E.C. "A Low-Carbohydrate, Ketogenic Diet for Type 2 Diabetes Mellitus," *Journal of General Internal Medicine,* 19(1S), 2004, p. 110.

Yancy, W.S., Jr., Olsen, M.K., and Guyton, J.R., et al. "A Low-Carbohydrate, Ketogenic Diet Versus a Low-Fat Diet to Treat Obesity and Hyperlipidemia," *Annals of Internal Medicine,* 140(10), 2004, pp. 769-777.

Yancy, W.S., Vernon, M.C., and Westman. E.C. "A Pilot Trial of a Low-Carbohydrate, Ketogenic Diet in Patients with Type 2 Diabetes," *Metabolic Syndrome and Related Disorders,* 1(3), 2003, pp. 239-243.

FIVE

Comparing the Low-Carb Diets

Bookstore shelves are full of titles about low-carb dieting. Each program takes a somewhat different approach, but in general they all advocate cutting carbs as part of an improved lifestyle that includes regular exercise. Chances are good that one of the programs will be right for you, but which one? The following descriptions highlight the main features of each plan and tell you how to learn more.

THE ATKINS NUTRITIONAL APPROACH

The original and perhaps still the best low-carb diet, the Atkins program is a four-phase approach. It begins with a two-week Induction period, where net carbs are limited to 20 grams a day. In Phase 2, Ongoing Weight Loss (OWL), daily net carbs are increased by 5 grams a week while weight loss continues. Phase 3, Pre-Maintenance, begins as your weight-loss goal nears. Daily net carbs are increased by 10 grams a week. Phase 4, Maintenance, begins when you are near or at your weight-loss goal. In this phase, even more net carbs are added back to your daily intake, until weight loss slows to a crawl or stops. This net carb level is your personal Atkins Carbohydrate Equilibrium (ACE)— the amount of net carbs you can take in each day without gaining weight. For most people, the ACE is at or under 60 net carb grams a day. If you want to increase your ACE, add more exercise.

The Atkins approach was first presented in the early 1970s and has been around and generating controversy ever since. Even so, every low-carb plan since then has been built on the pioneering work of the late Dr. Robert C. Atkins. Much of the controversy over Atkins—and all the other plans as well—stems from the mistaken idea that a low-carb diet means eating nothing but meat and eggs. Of course, this is and always has been far from the truth. Even during Induction, the most restrictive phase of Atkins, the plan calls for five daily servings of low-carb vegetables or salad. As carbs are added back, the Atkins approach encourages adding low-carb vegetables, low-carb fruits, and whole grains. The Atkins approach is also very firm on the subject of exercise—it's mandatory.

A major criticism of the Atkins diet is that it doesn't limit foods high in saturated fat and cholesterol, such as red meat, eggs, and cheese. The Atkins response is that foods high in saturated fat and cholesterol are indeed bad for you when eaten along with a high-carb diet full of refined grains. According to Atkins, when high-fat foods are eaten as part of a low-carb diet rich in vegetables and whole grains, blood cholesterol doesn't go up—in fact, it improves. Given the emphasis modern medicine places on cholesterol levels and a low-fat diet, this sounds impossible, yet recent research shows it may well be true. The Atkins approach has been extensively studied in recent years in carefully controlled experiments conducted by independent researchers. The results, presented in prestigious medical publications such as the *New England Journal of Medicine*, have been quite positive. The studies consistently show that when people following the standard reduced-calorie, low-fat approach to weight loss are compared to people following the Atkins low-carb approach, the amount of weight loss is about the same or greater on Atkins. More importantly, Atkins dieters generally show greater improvement in cholesterol levels and other measures of heart health such as blood pressure and blood sugar—even though they eat foods high in dietary fat (including saturated fat) and cholesterol.

Another criticism of the Atkins approach is that the Induction phase aims to cause ketosis (the presence of chemicals called ketones in the urine, a byproduct of burning fat as the body's primary fuel), which many doctors think is unhealthy. (Ketosis is discussed more on page 34.) Ketosis is generally safe for people who don't have kidney disease, but it's not necessary for successful weight loss on Atkins or any other low-carb diet. On the Atkins plan, those concerned about ketosis for any reason are encouraged to simply skip that phase and start instead with the lowest possible amount of carbs in the second phase, Ongoing Weight Loss. Yet another criticism—or misperception—is that doing Atkins means eating nothing but meat. Although the diet doesn't discourage these foods, they're not particularly encouraged either. In reality, the Atkins diet is quite varied and could be done easily even by someone who doesn't eat meat, poultry, or fish. It stresses eating a variety of protein foods, including lean meats, fish, eggs, dairy products, and tofu, and strongly stresses eating lots of low-carb vegetables. The diet also encourages nuts, beans, fruit, and whole grains, as long as portions are controlled.

To learn more about the Atkins approach, start with the classic volume *Dr. Atkins' New Diet Revolution* (Avon Books, 2001). This book is regularly updated to reflect the latest research on low-carb dieting, so get the most recent edition. To go beyond the basics, read *Atkins for Life* (St. Martin's Press, 2003) and *The Atkins Essentials* (Avon Books, 2004). For people with diabetes, *Atkins Diabetes Revolution* (William Morrow, 2004) is essential reading. The website for Atkins Nutritionals at www.atkins.com is an excellent source of free information, including many terrific low-carb recipes.

THE SOUTH BEACH DIET

Like Dr. Atkins, Dr. Arthur Agatston, the creator of the South Beach Diet, is a cardiologist whose concern for his patients led him to his approach. Although the author insists the South Beach diet is not a low-carbohydrate plan, it has striking resemblances to the Atkins approach. Among other similarities, the diet begins with a two-week period of strict low-carbing designed to help you get over cravings for sugar and other unhealthy foods, eliminate refined carbs from your diet, and kick-start weight loss. You don't count carbs or limit portions on the South Beach diet. You simply choose your foods from acceptable lists for each phase and limit or avoid the unacceptable foods. Your appetite is your guide to portion control.

The South Beach diet begins with Phase 1, a two-week period of major carb restriction. In Phase 1, you eat three full meals a day and two snacks, choosing from an extensive list of lean meats, seafood, eggs, cheese, nuts, beans, and lots of vegetables. High-carb foods such as bread, rice, pasta, and sweets of any sort are forbidden during this phase, as is fruit. In Phase 2, you start reintroducing carbs by having small amounts of fruit, dairy foods, whole grains, and other good carbs. The carbs are reintroduced slowly and carefully by choosing a single carbohydrate food—an apple or orange, for instance—and adding it to one daily meal for a week. If the food doesn't induce cravings for sugar or high-carb foods, it's OK for you, and you move on to trying an additional carbohydrate choice. During Phase 2, you discover which foods trigger cravings for you and learn to avoid them; likewise, you discover the foods you can enjoy without triggering cravings. Phase 2 goes on for as long as it takes for you to reach your weight-loss goal. By the end of Phase 2, you've added two to three servings a day of good carbohydrates. In Phase 3, you keep the weight off by continuing to follow the basic principles you learned in Phase 2, but you now use what you've learned to experiment with new foods.

The South Beach diet emphasizes good fats along with good carbs. The protein choices are limited to leaner meats, and the emphasis is more on fish and other low-fat choices. Good fats such as olive oil are encouraged; saturated fat is discouraged. Refined carbs such as cookies and white bread are out, as are foods high on the glycemic index such as french fries; whole grains are encouraged.

The South Beach diet has some scientific backup. In a study published in 2004 in *Archives of Internal Medicine*, the South Beach diet was compared to the National Cholesterol Education Program (NCEP) Step 2 diet (the standard low-fat, high-carb approach). Sixty overweight people were randomly assigned to one or the other diet. After three months, the South Beach dieters had lost more weight and had better cholesterol levels than the NCEP dieters.

For more information, read *The South Beach Diet* by Dr. Arthur Agatston (Rodale Books, 2003). The South Beach website at www.southbeachdiet.com has some useful free information and offers much more to paying subscribers.

THE HAMPTONS DIET

The Hampton's Diet was created by Dr. Fred Pescatore, a former associate of Dr. Robert C. Atkins. Dr. Pescatore combines the low-carb approach with a Mediterranean-style diet that emphasizes vegetables, fish, and consuming fats mostly in the form of monounsaturated oils such as olive oil. The diet also encourages lean proteins, whole grains, fruit, nuts, minimally processed foods, and minimal use of sugar alcohols, which are often used to artificially sweeten low-carb foods such as candy bars. Organic foods are suggested wherever possible. The Hamptons Diet also recommends using macadamia nut oil as the primary source of fat, because it is the most monounsaturated oil available. On this diet, there's no restrictive very-low-carb phase, so unrefined carbs and fruit are permitted from the start. You don't have to count carbs or measure portions. Foods are selected from lists organized in food pyramid form, making it easy to see what the most desirable choices are.

For more information, read *The Hamptons Diet* by Dr. Fred Pescatore (John Wiley & Sons, 2004) and check the website at www.hamptonsdiet.com.

THE CARBOHYDRATE ADDICT'S DIET

CAD, as the Carbohydrate Addict's Diet is called by those who follow it, has been popular since it was introduced in 1991 by the husband-and-wife team Richard F. Heller, Ph.D., and Rachel F. Heller, Ph.D. The underlying concept is that for many people, high insulin levels cause intense cravings for carbohydrate-rich foods, especially the unhealthy kind made with refined grains or lots of sugar. For those prone to carbohydrate addiction, the cravings can't be satisfied even by eating a high-carb food—their brain just doesn't send the "I'm full" signal. These people feel hungry all the time and have a very hard time controlling their desire for high-carb foods. The result is weight gain, along with high blood pressure, high cholesterol, diabetes, and other health problems. By controlling insulin levels with the Carbohydrate Addict's Diet, you control the cravings and can then start to eat better, lose weight, and improve your overall health.

The diet is designed to correct the high insulin problem and eliminate cravings with a two-pronged approach: timing and combining. You eat two low-carb meals a day (usually breakfast and lunch) consisting of equal portions of protein and nonstarchy vegetables. The third meal of the day (dinner for most people) is the "reward meal." For your reward meal, you eat a large green salad followed by a balanced meal that is one-third protein-rich foods, one-third nonstarchy vegetables, and one-third carbohydrate-rich foods. The high-carb food can be anything, including rice, potatoes, pasta, and even sweets or your favorite snack food. You don't have to measure portions or count carbs, and you can even go back for seconds. There are a couple of catches, though: If you want seconds, you have to maintain the third-third-third balance—in other words, no going back for more of just the high-carb foods—and the reward meal has to be fully eaten within one hour.

The CAD approach works quite well for many people, especially those who really miss eating carbohydrates and feel deprived if they don't have at least something starchy or sweet every day. Exercise is strongly recommended as part of the program. A criticism of the approach is that addicts shouldn't be encouraged to use the substance they're addicted to, and that someone who can't control cravings for carbohydrates should stay away from them as much as possible. Another criticism is that it's all too easy to cheat on the reward meal and eat excessively large portions. By allowing junk foods, the diet lets you eat unhealthy trans fats and large amounts of salt.

The diet was first introduced in *The Carbohydrate Addict's Diet* by Dr. Rachael F. Heller and Dr. Richard F. Heller (E. P. Dutton, 1991). Other volumes since then have expanded and updated the approach, particularly *The Carbohydrate Addict's Lifespan Program* (E. P. Dutton, 1997) and *The Carbohydrate Addict's Healthy Heart Program* (Ballantine Books, 1999). The website at www.carbohydrateaddicts.com has some useful information.

PROTEIN POWER

Although a low-carb diet doesn't have to also be a high-protein diet, the Protein Power approach is. Michael Eades, M.D., and his wife Mary Dan Eades, M.D., specialize in weight loss and devised the program based on their experience with their patients. The diet's basic premise is that an adequate amount of high-quality protein should be the core of every meal and that carbohydrate intake should be limited. Like Atkins, the diet has phases. Phase I is Intervention, where carbohydrates are limited to 30 grams or less a day. This phase continues for at least three to four weeks and may go on much longer if you are seriously overweight. Phase II, Transition, slowly adds more carbohydrates, but limits them to 55 grams a day or less. This allows weight loss to continue until you reach your goal. At that point, Phase III, Maintenance begins. Carbohydrates are increased just enough to keep you at your goal weight.

Protein Power is well grounded in the science of carbohydrate metabolism. As in the Atkins diet, fiber in carbohy-drates doesn't count—in Protein Power the net carbs count is called the effective carbohydrate content. A major criticism of the Protein Power diet is that exercise gets very little attention.

To learn more, read *Protein Power* (Bantam, 1997) and *The Protein Power Lifeplan* (Warner Books, 2001).

SUGAR BUSTERS!™

The Sugar Busters! approach is deceptively simple: Cut out the sugar, refined carbs, and starchy vegetables and you'll lose weight and improve your health. The main culprit here is refined sugar; the main goal is to control insulin production. Beneath the simplicity is sound scientific reasoning and a good use of the glycemic index to help you choose better foods. The diet doesn't count carbs or portions and doesn't outline a specific program or steps to take. The recommendation is simply to cut back on carbs, especially refined grains and sugar. Weight loss and better health will almost certainly follow.

Sugar Busters! by H. Leighton Steward; Sam S. Andrews, M.D.; Morrison C. Bethea, M.D.; and Luis A. Balart, M.D., is the original book (Ballantine Books, 1995). The basic idea is expanded in *The New Sugar Busters* by the same authors (Ballantine Books, 2002). More information can be found at the website, www.sugarbusters.com.

THE ZONE

The Zone diet, developed by Barry Sears, Ph.D., is based on the concept that eating a lot of refined carbohydrates raises insulin levels, leading to weight gain. Lower insulin levels lead to weight loss and better health. The solution is to keep your insulin levels in the Zone with a diet that's 40 percent unrefined, low-glycemic carbohydrates, 30 percent protein, and 30 percent fat. This diet is conceptually sound and balanced, but it takes a fair amount of attention to detail and planning. The overall goal at each meal is to have the 40/30/30 balance, which isn't always easy to achieve. Foods are categorized into blocks: a protein block is a portion that contains 7 grams of protein, a carbohydrate block contains 9 grams, and a fat block contains 1.5 grams. Based on a simple calculation of your daily needs for all three nutrients, you determine how many blocks of each food type to eat at each meal. A typical meal would include four carbohydrate blocks—four portions containing 36 carb grams in total. Carbohydrates are preferably chosen from moderate- to low-carb vegetables, whole grains, and fruit. For example, the meal could include 1 cup cooked broccoli (10 carb grams) and half a cup of cooked barley (22 carb grams). In addition, the typical meal would include three protein blocks and three fat blocks (preferably not saturated fat). When you add up the calories, though, that turns out to be a backdoor way of getting you to limit your intake, and with 40 percent of calories coming from carbohydrates, the diet isn't really low-carb. It relies more on portion control, which usually leads to weight loss but can leave you hungry. Many athletes swear by the Zone approach, however, and the balanced approach works well for some people.

To learn more, read *The Zone* (ReganBooks, 1995) or any of the follow-up titles, such as *Mastering the Zone* (Regan-Books, 1997). The website at www.zoneperfect.com has a lot of very good information.

WEIGHT WATCHERS

Officially, Weight Watchers is strongly opposed to low-carb dieting. In reality, however, the Core Plan program, introduced in 2004, is a back-door approach to low-carbing. For years, Weight Watchers has used a low-fat, reduced-calorie approach based on a point system. It's an effective and fairly flexible approach for people who can handle measuring their portions, counting calories and fat grams, and tracking their daily and weekly points. In the face of competition from the low-carbohydrate lifestyle, however, which doesn't require such a meticulous, plan-in-advance approach, Weight Watchers designed the Core Plan. Instead of careful point counting and portion control paticipants select their foods from limited lists of protein choices, vegetables, grains, and so on, and simply eat enough of those foods to satisfy their appetites. The emphasis is on whole foods that are high in volume but low in energy density—in other words, foods that fill you up without a lot of calories. What that comes down to is that you're allowed unrestricted amounts of lean meats, fish and seafood, poultry, and soy foods, fresh fruits and vegetables, and plain nonfat or low-fat dairy products. Whole grains and the few allowed breakfast cereals are limited to one serving daily, and dietrary fat is kept low. What's conspicuously missing from the allowed lists are almost all high-carb foods. Bread, french fries, dried fruits, snack foods, almost all breakfast cereals, and pretty much anything made with white flour or sugar are out. It that sounds very familiar, it's becauce the lists are actually quite similar to the allowed foods on the mid-level stages of Atkins or South Beach. A major difference is that the Core Plan strongly discourages dietary fat, limiting it to just a couple of teaspoons of healthy vegetable oils each day and recommending fat-free salad dressings and nonfat and low-fat dairy products. The plan allows a few splurges balanced out over a week, including things like real butter, mayonnaise, and full-fat cheese in small amounts.

The structured, fee-based approach of Weight Watchers, which includes regular group meetings (in-person or online) and personalized counseling, is helpful for many people. The Core Plan approach combines the flexibility and simplicity of low-carbing (even if they don't call it that) with the supportive Weight Watchers environment.

To learn more about the Weight Watchers approach and the Core Plan program, contact a local Weight Watchers center (check your phone book) or go to www.WeightWatchers.com. The website doesn't provide much for free but has a lot of good information, recipes, and advice for subscribers.

THE ROSEDALE DIET

Another diet that's low-carb even though it says it's not, the Rosedale Diet is based on the idea that controlling the hormone leptin, which plays an important role in making you feel both hungry and satiated, can help you lose weight. Overweight people produce too much leptin, to the point that their bodies become desensitized to it and they don't respond to the hormone when it sends the "stop eating" order. Eating carbohydrates, especially refined carbs, makes leptin levels soar, while good fats suppresses leptin production. The Rosedale approach works by sharply restricting carbs, keeping protein intake moderate (50 to 70 grams a day), and making sure you get plenty of good fats. The diet lowers leptin levels—and when leptin goes down and your body becomes more responsive to it, weight comes off without hunger.

Dr. Ron Rosedale bases his plan on the exciting new research on leptin that has been appearing since 1995—the diet has a strong scientific basis. Most people begin by spending three weeks on Level 1. During this phase, you eat virtually no carbs, but you do eat plenty of high-fiber vegetables, moderate amounts of protein, and foods that are high in good fat, such as fish, nuts, and avocados. In Level 2, you move on to adding back some carbohydrates such as fruit and additional protein sources such as cheese and beef. You don't count calories, carb grams, or portions. Mild exercise—just 15 minutes a day—is strongly recommended.

To learn more about this diet, read *The Rosedale Diet* (HarperCollins, 2004) and check the website at www.rose dalemetabolics.com.

SIX

How to Use These Tables

The tables in this section provide nutritional information for well over 2,500 frequently eaten foods. They are organized alphabetically by broad food categories (a list can be found in the Table of Contents). Within each food category, they are organized alphabetically, usually by the type of food. For instance, in the vegetables table, the listing begins with acorn squash and ends with zucchini. In some cases, where a brand name is the most common name for a food, the brand name is listed instead (Oreo® instead of chocolate crème-filled wafer cookie). For each individual entry, the food is listed, followed in many cases by the brand name. Moving horizontally, the usual serving size is given first, followed by carbohydrates, fiber, net carbs, calories, protein, and fat. Where reduced-carb products are available, they are listed in a separate table. In some cases, those tables have an additional column for sugar alcohol.

All food component measurements (carbohydrates, fiber, sugar alcohols, net carbohydrates, protein, and fat) are given in grams. In most cases serving sizes are based on standard portions used by nutritionists and are given in standard kitchen measurements (1 cup, for example) or by the piece (one medium apple). For processed foods, however, the serving size is whatever the manufacturer has designated on the food facts label (3 cookies, for example).

The information in these tables comes from the U.S. Department of Agriculture Nutrient Database (2004 release), food manufacturers, and fast food restaurants. It's as accurate as possible, but food manufacturers and restaurants sometimes stop offering a product or modify it in ways that can change the nutritional content. Always read the food facts label carefully for the most current information.

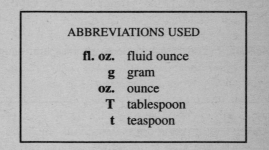

ABBREVIATIONS USED

fl. oz. fluid ounce

g gram

oz. ounce

T tablespoon

t teaspoon

BAKED PRODUCTS: BROWNIES, CAKES, DOUGHNUTS, AND PIES

Let's face it: It's hard to stay away from bakery goodies such as doughnuts. But do you have to cut out cake completely? Can you never bite into a brownie or devour a doughnut? No. Just be aware that they're high in refined carbs, often contain undesirable trans fats, and have very little in the way of redeeming nutrition. Just thinking about that should help you turn to better choices! Save the baked goods for special treats like birthdays and do your best to avoid them at other times.

This section includes snack cakes. Cookies, bread, breakfast pastries, and other snack foods are in separate sections.

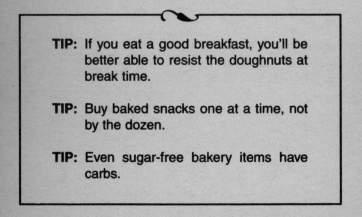

TIP: If you eat a good breakfast, you'll be better able to resist the doughnuts at break time.

TIP: Buy baked snacks one at a time, not by the dozen.

TIP: Even sugar-free bakery items have carbs.

Food	Serving size	Carbohy-drates	Fiber	Net Carbs	Calories	Protein	Fat
Angel food cake	1 oz.	16	0	16	72	2	0
Apple fritter, Dunkin' Donuts	1 fritter	41	1	40	300	4	14
Brownie	1 2x2 brownie	12	0	12	112	2	7
Boston cream pie	1 slice	40	1	39	232	2	8
Cheesecake, no-bake	1 slice	35	2	33	271	5	7
Chocolate cake	1 slice	51	2	49	340	5	14
Coffeecake, crumb topping	1 slice	29	1	28	263	4	15
Coffee roll, Dunkin' Donuts	1 roll	33	1	32	270	4	14
Cruller, glazed	1 cruller	24	0	24	169	1	8
Cruller, Dunkin' Donuts	1 cruller	17	1	16	150	2	8
Danish pastry, apple, Dunkin' Donuts	1 pastry	36	0	36	250	4	10
Danish pastry, cheese	1 pastry	26	1	25	266	6	16
Danish pastry, fruit	1 pastry	34	1	33	263	4	13
Ding Dongs	1 cake	45	2	43	368	3	19
Doughnut, Bavarian Kreme, Dunkin' Donuts	1 doughnut	30	1	29	210	3	9

Food	Serving size	Carbohy-drates	Fiber	Net Carbs	Calories	Protein	Fat
Doughnut, Boston Kreme, Dunkin' Donuts	1 doughnut	36	1	35	240	3	9
Doughnut, cake	1 doughnut	23	1	22	198	2	11
Doughnut, cake, Dunkin' Donuts	1 doughnut	28	1	27	300	4	19
Doughnut, chocolate frosted, Dunkin' Donuts	1 doughnut	29	1	28	200	3	9
Doughnut, crème	1 doughnut	25	1	24	307	5	21
Doughnut, glazed	1 doughnut	23	1	22	192	2	10
Doughnut, glazed, Dunkin' Donuts	1 doughnut	25	1	24	180	3	8
Doughnut, jelly	1 doughnut	33	1	32	289	5	16
Doughnut, jelly, Dunkin' Donuts	1 doughnut	32	1	31	210	3	8
Doughnut, sugared	1 doughnut	23	1	22	192	2	10
Éclair, chocolate	1 éclair	24	1	23	262	6	16
Éclair, Dunkin' Donuts	1 éclair	39	1	38	270	3	11
Fruitcake	1 slice	27	2	25	139	1	4
Gingerbread	1 slice	36	0	36	263	3	12
Hostess snack cake	1 cake	45	2	43	368	3	19

Food	Serving size	Carbohy-drates	Fiber	Net Carbs	Calories	Protein	Fat
Munchkin, glazed, Dunkin' Donuts	5 pieces	27	1	26	200	3	9
Munchkin, jelly, Dunkin' Donuts	5 pieces	30	1	29	210	3	9
Pie, apple	1 slice	56	0	56	411	4	20
Pie, banana cream	1 slice	47	1	46	387	6	20
Pie, blueberry	1 slice	44	1	43	290	2	13
Pie, cherry	1 slice	69	0	69	486	5	22
Pie, chocolate cream	1 slice	38	2	36	344	3	22
Pie, lemon meringue	1 slice	50	0	50	362	5	16
Pie, peach	1 slice	39	1	38	261	2	12
Pie, pecan	1 slice	65	4	61	452	5	21
Pie, pumpkin	1 slice	41	0	41	316	7	14
Pineapple upside-down cake	1 slice	58	1	57	367	4	14
Pound cake	1 slice	15	0	15	116	2	6
Sponge cake	1 slice	23	0	23	110	2	1
Strudel, apple	2½ oz.	29	2	27	195	2	8
Yellow cake	1 slice	36	0	36	245	4	10

BEANS AND PEAS

Versatile, inexpensive, and very low in fat, beans and peas are a good source of vegetable protein. They're also rich in iron, calcium, potassium, and B vitamins. Even when you deduct the large amounts of fiber per portion, however, beans and peas are still a little on the high side for net carbs. You can definitely enjoy them as part of a varied low-carb diet, but be aware of portion size. Fortunately, beans and peas are also very filling, so a small serving goes a long way as a side dish or as an interesting and healthful addition to salads, soups, and stews.

Watch out for baked beans—the added sugar in them means that a single half-cup serving generally contains between 20 and 30 net carbs. Similarly, beans and peas in sauces will almost always have extra net carbs.

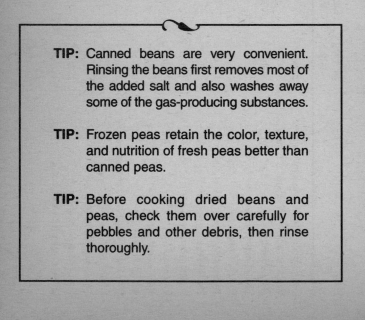

TIP: Canned beans are very convenient. Rinsing the beans first removes most of the added salt and also washes away some of the gas-producing substances.

TIP: Frozen peas retain the color, texture, and nutrition of fresh peas better than canned peas.

TIP: Before cooking dried beans and peas, check them over carefully for pebbles and other debris, then rinse thoroughly.

Food	Serving size	Carbohy-drates	Fiber	Net Carbs	Calories	Protein	Fat
Baked beans, barbecue, Bush's	½ cup	32	6	26	160	6	1
Baked beans, bold & spicy, Bush's	½ cup	24	5	19	120	6	0.5
Baked beans, Boston recipe, Bush's	½ cup	32	6	26	170	6	1.5
Baked beans, country style, Bush's	½ cup	33	7	26	170	7	1
Baked beans, original, B&M	½ cup	30	6	24	140	6	1
Baked beans, original, Bush's	½ cup	29	7	22	150	7	1
Baked beans, original, Van Camp's	½ cup	30	6	24	140	7	1
Baked beans, vegetarian, Heinz	½ cup	27	5	22	140	6	0.5
Black beans, canned	1 cup	41	15	26	227	15	1
Black-eyed peas, canned	1 cup	32	8	24	185	11	1
Butter beans, canned	½ cup	39	13	26	108	8	1
Chick peas (garbanzo beans), canned	1 cup	45	13	32	269	15	4
Chili beans, canned, Bush's	½ cup	20	6	14	120	6	1
Cranberry beans, canned	1 cup	39	16	23	216	14	1
Fava beans, cooked	1 cup	33	9	24	187	13	1
Great northern beans, canned	1 cup	37	12	25	209	15	1
Hummus	1 T	2	1	1	23	1	1

Food	Serving size	Carbohy-drates	Fiber	Net Carbs	Calories	Protein	Fat
Lentils, cooked	1 cup	40	16	24	230	18	1
Lima beans, baby, cooked	1 cup	40	9	31	209	12	1
Mung beans, cooked	1 cup	39	15	24	212	14	1
Navy beans, canned	1 cup	54	13	41	296	20	1
Peas, green, canned	1 cup	21	7	14	117	8	0.5
Peas, green, frozen, boiled	½ cup	11	4	7	62	4	0
Peas, split, cooked	1 cup	41	16	25	231	16	1
Pink beans, cooked	1 cup	47	9	38	252	15	1
Pinto beans, canned	1 cup	37	11	26	206	12	2
Pork and beans, Campbell's	½ cup	27	7	20	140	6	1
Refried beans, canned	1 cup	39	13	26	237	14	3
Refried beans, Ortega	½ cup	25	9	16	150	8	2.5
Refried beans, cheese, Old El Paso	½ cup	18	6	12	130	7	3.5
Refried beans, fat-free, Old El Paso	½ cup	17	6	11	100	6	0
Refried beans, green chilies, Old El Paso	½ cup	19	6	13	100	6	0.5
Refried beans, traditional, Old El Paso	½ cup	17	6	11	100	6	0.5
White beans, canned	1 cup	58	13	45	307	19	1

BEEF, VEAL, AND LAMB

Beef has zero carbs, making it a delicious and convenient addition to any low-carb diet. Although veal and lamb are less popular than beef, they too are flavorful and satisfying, with zero carbs. Even though beef, veal, and lamb themselves have no carbs, watch out for breading, stuffings, and condiments such as ketchup and steak sauces—those extra carbs can add up.

To store beef, veal, and lamb safely, refrigerate them as soon as possible after purchasing. The USDA recommends cooking beef until it is at least medium rare, or 160° F in the middle; for veal, the recommendation is also 160° F; for lamb, the recommendation is 145° F.

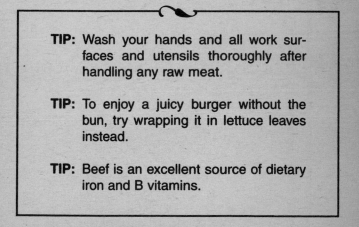

TIP: Wash your hands and all work surfaces and utensils thoroughly after handling any raw meat.

TIP: To enjoy a juicy burger without the bun, try wrapping it in lettuce leaves instead.

TIP: Beef is an excellent source of dietary iron and B vitamins.

Food	Serving size	Carbohy-drates	Fiber	Net Carbs	Calories	Protein	Fat
BEEF (all portions are cooked)							
Bottom round, roasted	3 oz.	0	0	0	199	23	11
Bottom sirloin roast	3 oz.	0	0	0	184	24	9
Breakfast strips	3 strips	0.5	0	0.5	153	11	9
Brisket, braised	3 oz.	0	0	0	189	27	8
Chuck roast	3 oz.	0	0	0	206	21	13
Chuck steak, braised	3 oz.	0	0	0	231	23	15
Corned beef brisket	3 oz.	0	0	0	213	15	16
Flank steak, braised	3 oz.	0	0	0	224	23	14
Ground, 5% fat, broiled	3 oz.	0	0	0	145	22	6
Ground, 10% fat, broiled	3 oz.	0	0	0	184	22	10
Ground, 15% fat, broiled	3 oz.	0	0	0	213	22	13
Ground, 20% fat, broiled	3 oz.	0	0	0	230	22	15
Ground, 25% fat, broiled	3 oz.	0	0	0	236	22	16
Porterhouse, broiled	3 oz.	0	0	0	264	20	20
Rib eye roast	3 oz.	0	0	0	333	14	28
Rib eye steak, broiled	3 oz.	0	0	0	261	21	19

Food	Serving size	Carbohy-drates	Fiber	Net Carbs	Calories	Protein	Fat
Ribs, prime, roasted	3 oz.	0	0	0	342	19	29
Ribs, short, braised	3 oz.	0	0	0	400	18	36
Round, bottom, braised	3 oz.	0	0	0	220	25	13
Round, eye, roasted	3 oz.	0	0	0	137	24	4
Round, top, broiled	3 oz.	0	0	0	175	26	7
Sirloin, top, broiled	3 oz.	0	0	0	229	24	14
Skirt steak, broiled	3 oz.	0	0	0	217	20	15
T-bone steak, broiled	3 oz.	0	0	0	239	21	17
Tenderloin, broiled	3 oz.	0	0	0	230	22	15

VEAL (all portions are cooked)

Food	Serving size	Carbohy-drates	Fiber	Net Carbs	Calories	Protein	Fat
Chop, loin, braised	3 oz.	0	0	0	284	30	17
Ground, broiled	3 oz.	0	0	0	172	24	8
Liver, braised	3 oz.	0	0	0	165	22	7
Rib, roasted	3 oz.	0	0	0	251	24	13
Stew, braised	3 oz.	0	0	0	188	35	4

Food	Serving size	Carbohy-drates	Fiber	Net Carbs	Calories	Protein	Fat
LAMB (all portions are cooked)							
Ground, broiled	3 oz.	0	0	0	241	21	17
Leg, roasted	3 oz.	0	0	0	153	24	6
Loin, roasted	3 oz.	0	0	0	172	23	8
Rib, broiled	3 oz.	0	0	0	289	20	23
Shoulder, arm, braised	3 oz.	0	0	0	237	30	12
Shoulder, arm, broiled	3 oz.	0	0	0	239	21	17
Shoulder, blade, braised	3 oz.	0	0	0	245	28	14
Shoulder, blade, broiled	3 oz.	0	0	0	179	22	10

BEVERAGES

You might be able to cut a lot of carbs from your diet simply by changing what you drink. Switching from a regular beer to low-carb beer, for instance, could save 7 net carb grams a serving. And switching from regular cola to diet cola saves a whopping 27 net carb grams a serving. Ditto for other popular beverages such as orange juice and sports drinks. Cut back on the high-carb drinks, dilute them with water or club soda—2 ounces of OJ in 6 ounces of seltzer makes a very refreshing low-carb drink—or choose sugar-free versions.

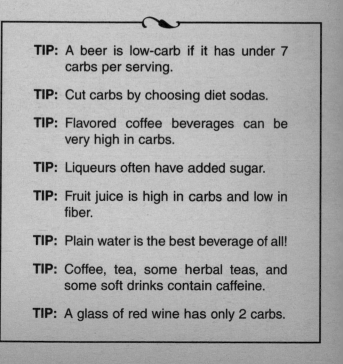

TIP: A beer is low-carb if it has under 7 carbs per serving.

TIP: Cut carbs by choosing diet sodas.

TIP: Flavored coffee beverages can be very high in carbs.

TIP: Liqueurs often have added sugar.

TIP: Fruit juice is high in carbs and low in fiber.

TIP: Plain water is the best beverage of all!

TIP: Coffee, tea, some herbal teas, and some soft drinks contain caffeine.

TIP: A glass of red wine has only 2 carbs.

BEER AND MALT BEVERAGES

Food	Serving size	Carbohy-drates	Fiber	Net Carbs	Calories	Protein	Fat
Bacardi Silver	12 fl. oz.	38	0	38	220	0	0
Beer	12 fl. oz.	13	0	13	146	0	0
Beer, light	12 fl. oz.	5	0	5	99	0	0
Bud Dry	12 fl. oz.	8	0	8	130	1	0
Bud Ice	12 fl. oz.	9	0	9	148	1	0
Bud Ice Light	12 fl. oz.	7	0	7	110	1	0
Bud Light	12 fl. oz.	7	0	7	110	1	0
Budweiser	12 fl. oz.	11	0	11	143	1	0
Busch	12 fl. oz.	10	0	10	133	1	0
Busch Ice	12 fl. oz.	13	0	13	172	1	0
Busch Light	12 fl. oz.	8	0	8	110	1	0
Busch NA (no alcohol)	12 fl. oz.	13	0	13	60	1	0
Colt 45 malt liquor	12 fl. oz.	11	0	11	159	1	0
Coors Extra Gold	12 fl. oz.	11	0	11	147	1	0
Coors Light	12 fl. oz.	5	0	5	105	1	0
Coors nonalcoholic	12 fl. oz.	14	0	14	73	1	0

Food	Serving size	Carbohy-drates	Fiber	Net Carbs	Calories	Protein	Fat
Coors Original	12 fl. oz.	11	0	11	148	1	0
George Killian's Irish Red	12 fl. oz.	14	0	14	163	2	0
Hurricane	12 fl. oz.	10	0	10	158	1	0
Keystone	12 fl. oz.	6	0	6	122	1	0
Keystone Ice	12 fl. oz.	5	0	5	129	1	0
Keystone Light	12 fl. oz.	5	0	5	100	1	0
King Cobra	12 fl. oz.	12	0	12	166	1	0
Lowenbrau dark	12 fl. oz.	14	0	14	158	1	0
Malt beverage, nonalcoholic	12 fl. oz.	48	0	48	214	1	0
Michelob	12 fl. oz.	13	0	13	155	1	0
Michelob Amber Bock	12 fl. oz.	15	0	15	166	1	0
Michelob Black & Tan	12 fl. oz.	16	0	16	168	2	0
Michelob Golden Draft	12 fl. oz.	14	0	14	152	1	0
Michelob Golden Draft Light	12 fl. oz.	7	0	7	110	1	0
Michelob Hefeweizen	12 fl. oz.	17	0	17	176	3	0
Michelob Honey Lager	12 fl. oz.	18	0	18	175	2	0
Michelob Light	12 fl. oz.	12	0	12	134	1	0

Food	Serving size	Carbohy-drates	Fiber	Net Carbs	Calories	Protein	Fat
Michelob Ultra	12 fl. oz.	2	0	2	92	0	0
Miller	12 fl. oz.	13	0	13	150	1	0
Miller Lite	12 fl. oz.	3	0	3	96	1	0
Miller Lite Ice	12 fl. oz.	4	0	4	113	0	0
Natural Ice	12 fl. oz.	9	0	9	157	1	0
Natural Light	12 fl. oz.	7	0	7	110	1	0
O'Doul's (nonalcoholic)	12 fl. oz.	13	0	13	70	1	0
O'Doul's Amber (nonalcoholic)	12 fl. oz.	18	0	18	90	2	0
Rock Green Light	12 fl. oz.	2	0	2	83	1	0
Rolling Rock	12 fl. oz.	7	0	7	120	2	0
Sam Adams Light	12 fl. oz.	8	0	8	125	1	0
Samuel Adams	12 fl. oz.	17	0	17	159	0	0
Zima	12 fl. oz.	21	0	21	185	0	0
Zima Citrus	12 fl. oz.	21	0	21	185	0	0

REDUCED-CARB PRODUCTS

Food	Serving size	Carbohy-drates	Fiber	Net Carbs	Calories	Protein	Fat
Accel	12 fl. oz.	2.4	0	2.4	89	0	0
Amstel Light	12 fl. oz.	5	0	5	95	0	0
Aspen Edge	12 fl. oz.	2.6	0	2.6	94	0	0
Bud Ice Light	12 fl. oz.	6.5	0	6.5	112	0	0
Bud Light	12 fl. oz.	6.6	0	6.6	110	0	0
Busch Light	12 fl. oz.	6.7	0	6.7	110	0	0
Coastal Light	12 fl. oz.	3.9	0	3.9	95	0	0
Coors Light	12 fl. oz.	5	0	5	102	0	0
Corona Light	12 fl. oz.	5	0	5	105	0	0
Genny Light	12 fl. oz.	5.5	0	5.5	96	0	0
I.C. Light	12 fl. oz.	2.9	0	2.9	96	0	0
Iron City Light	12 fl. oz.	2.8	0	2.8	95	0	0
Keystone Light	12 fl. oz.	5	0	5	104	0	0
Labatt Select	12 fl. oz.	2.5	0	2.5	99	0	0
Michelob Ultra	12 fl. oz.	2.6	0	2.6	95	0	0
Mike's Light Lemonade	12 fl. oz.	2	0	2	84	0	0

Food	Serving size	Carbohy-drates	Fiber	Net Carbs	Calories	Protein	Fat
Miller Lite	12 fl. oz.	3.2	0	3.2	96	0	0
Milwaukee's Best Light	12 fl. oz.	3.5	0	3.5	98	0	0
Molson Ultra	12 fl. oz.	2.5	0	2.5	97	0	0
Natural Light	12 fl. oz.	3.2	0	3.2	95	0	0
Rhinebecker Extra	12 fl. oz.	2.5	0	2.5	106	0	0
Rock Green Light	12 fl. oz.	2.6	0	2.6	92	0	0
Thin Ice	12 fl. oz.	1	0	1	90	0	0
CARBONATED DRINKS							
A&W cream soda	12 fl. oz.	46	0	0	180	0	0
A&W diet cream soda	12 fl. oz.	0	0	0	0	0	0
Barq's root beer	12 fl. oz.	30	0	30	111	0	0
Canada Dry Diet Ginger Ale	12 fl. oz.	0	0	0	0	0	0
Canada Dry Ginger Ale	12 fl. oz.	38	0	38	135	0	0
Cherry Coke	12 fl. oz.	28	0	28	104	0	0
Club soda	12 fl. oz.	0	0	0	0	0	0
Coca Cola Classic	12 fl. oz.	27	0	27	97	0	0

Food	Serving size	Carbohy-drates	Fiber	Net Carbs	Calories	Protein	Fat
Coca Cola Classic caffeine-free	12 fl. oz.	27	0	27	97	0	0
Cola, generic	12 fl. oz.	39	0	39	152	0	0
Cream soda, generic	12 fl. oz.	49	0	49	189	0	0
Diet Barq's root beer	12 fl. oz.	0	0	0	1	0	0
Diet Cherry Coke	12 fl. oz.	0	0	0	0	0	0
Diet Coke	12 fl. oz.	0	0	0	1	0	0
Diet Coke caffeine-free	12 fl. oz.	0	0	0	1	0	0
Diet cola, with aspartame	12 fl. oz.	0	0	0	4	0	0
Diet Dr. Pepper	12 fl. oz.	0	0	0	0	0	0
Diet Mello Yello	12 fl. oz.	0	0	0	3	0	0
Diet Minute Maid Orange	12 fl. oz.	0	0	0	2	0	0
Diet Mr. Pibb	12 fl. oz.	0	0	0	1	0	0
Diet Pepsi	12 fl. oz.	0	0	0	0	0	0
Diet RC Cola	12 fl. oz.	0	0	0	0	0	0
Diet Sprite	12 fl. oz.	0	0	0	2	0	0
Dr. Pepper	12 fl. oz.	41	0	41	162	0	0
Fanta	12 fl. oz.	32	0	32	117	0	0

Food	Serving size	Carbohy-drates	Fiber	Net Carbs	Calories	Protein	Fat
Fresca	12 fl. oz.	0	0	0	2	0	0
Ginger ale, generic	12 fl. oz.	32	0	32	124	0	0
Grape, generic	12 fl. oz.	42	0	42	160	0	0
Inca Kola	12 fl. oz.	26	0	26	96	0	0
Mello Yello	12 fl. oz.	32	0	32	118	0	0
Minute Maid	12 fl. oz.	31	0	31	115	0	0
Mountain Dew	12 fl. oz.	31	0	31	110	0	0
Mr. Pibb	12 fl. oz.	26	0	26	97	0	0
Pepsi	12 fl. oz.	41	0	41	150	0	0
RC Cola	12 fl. oz.	42	0	42	120	0	0
Root beer, generic	12 fl. oz.	39	0	39	152	0	0
7-Up	12 fl. oz.	39	0	39	150	0	0
Shasta	12 fl. oz.	44	0	44	175	0	0
Shasta diet	12 fl. oz.	0	0	0	0	0	0
Sprite	12 fl. oz.	26	0	26	96	0	0
Sunkist diet orange soda	12 fl. oz.	0	0	0	0	0	0
Sunkist orange soda	12 fl. oz.	53	0	53	195	0	0

Food	Serving size	Carbohy- drates	Fiber	Net Carbs	Calories	Protein	Fat
Surge	12 fl. oz.	31	0	31	116	0	0
Tab	12 fl. oz.	0	0	0	1	0	0
Tonic water	12 fl. oz.	32	0	32	124	0	0

COFFEE AND COFFEE BEVERAGES

Food	Serving size	Carbohy- drates	Fiber	Net Carbs	Calories	Protein	Fat
Café au lait, Starbucks	16 fl. oz.	11	0	11	140	8	8
Caffè Americano, Starbucks	16 fl. oz.	3	0	3	15	1	0
Caffè latte, Starbucks	16 fl. oz.	21	0	21	260	14	14
Caffè mocha, whipped cream, Starbucks	16 fl. oz.	42	2	40	400	13	22
Cappucino, Dunkin' Donuts	10 fl. oz.	7	0	7	80	4	5
Cappucino, Starbucks	16 fl. oz.	13	0	13	150	8	8
Caramel Frappucino Blended Coffee, Starbucks	16 fl. oz.	57	0	57	280	5	3.5
Caramel Macchiato, Starbucks	16 fl. oz.	37	0	37	310	12	7
Caramel Mocha, Starbucks	16 fl. oz.	61	2	59	370	13	11
Caramel Swirl Latte, Dunkin' Donuts	10 fl. oz.	36	0	36	230	8	6
Coffee, brewed	8 fl. oz.	1	0	1	5	0	0

Food	Serving size	Carbohy-drates	Fiber	Net Carbs	Calories	Protein	Fat
Coffee, brewed, decaf	8 fl. oz.	1	0	1	5	0	0
Coffee Coolatta, Dunkin' Donuts	16 fl. oz.	42	0	42	210	4	4
Coffee Frappucino Blended Coffee, Starbucks	16 fl. oz.	52	0	52	260	5	3.5
Coffee Frappucino Light Blended Coffee, Starbucks	16 fl. oz.	30	3	27	150	7	1
Coffee, instant	8 fl. oz.	1	0	1	5	0	0
Coffee, instant, Café Francais	8 fl. oz.	7	0	7	62	0	0
Coffee, instant, decaf	8 fl. oz.	1	0	1	4	0	0
Coffee, instant, French vanilla	8 fl. oz.	10	0	10	65	0	0
Coffee, instant, Suisse mocha	8 fl. oz.	9	0	9	57	0	0
Eggnog latte, Starbucks	16 fl. oz.	41	0	41	410	17	20
Espresso	2 fl. oz.	1	0	1	0	0	0
Espresso Frappucino, Starbucks	16 fl. oz.	46	0	46	230	5	3
Espresso macchiato, Starbucks	2 fl. oz.	1	0	2	8	0	0
Frappucino Blended Coffee, Starbucks	16 fl. oz.	72	0	72	340	6	3.5
Frappucino Light Blended Coffee, Starbucks	16 fl. oz.	49	0	49	230	7	1

Food	Serving size	Carbohydrates	Fiber	Net Carbs	Calories	Protein	Fat
Latte, Dunkin' Donuts	10 fl. oz.	10	0	10	120	6	6
Mocha Swirl Latte, Dunkin' Donuts	10 fl. oz.	37	0	37	230	6	7

DISTILLED SPIRITS AND MIXED DRINKS

Food	Serving size	Carbohydrates	Fiber	Net Carbs	Calories	Protein	Fat
Amaretto	1 fl. oz.	17	0	17	110	0	0
Bailey's Irish Cream	1 fl. oz.	5	0	5	95	0	5
Benedictine	1 fl. oz.	5	0	5	90	0	0
Bloody mary	6 fl. oz.	9	0	9	42	2	0
Brandy	1 fl. oz.	0	0	0	75	0	0
Chambord	1 fl. oz.	11	0	11	103	0	0
Chartreuse	1 fl. oz.	7	0	7	100	0	0
Cointreau	1 fl. oz.	7	0	7	100	0	0
Cosmopolitan	6 fl. oz.	16	0	16	243	0	0
Crème de menthe	1.5 fl. oz.	21	0	21	186	0	0
Daiquiri	2 fl. oz.	4	0	4	112	0	0
Drambuie	1 fl. oz.	9	0	9	105	0	0
Frangelico	1 fl. oz.	9	0	9	80	0	0

Food	Serving size	Carbohy-drates	Fiber	Net Carbs	Calories	Protein	Fat
Gin	1.5 fl. oz.	0	0	0	97	0	0
Grand Marnier	1 fl. oz.	7	0	7	100	0	0
Irish coffee	6 fl. oz.	8	0	8	210	0	0
Kahlua	1 fl. oz.	11	0	11	98	0	0
Mai tai	6 fl. oz.	17	0	17	260	0	0
Martini	6 fl. oz.	1	0	1	160	0	0
Midori	1 fl. oz.	11	0	11	80	0	0
Piña colada	4.5 fl. oz.	32	0	32	252	1	3
Rum	1.5 fl. oz.	0	0	0	97	0	0
Screwdriver	6 fl. oz.	20	0	20	180	0	0
Tequila	1 fl. oz.	16	0	16	65	0	0
Tequila sunrise	6 fl. oz.	14	0	14	190	0	0
Tia Maria	1 fl. oz.	9	0	9	90	0	0
Triple Sec	1 fl. oz.	4	0	4	80	0	0
Vodka	1.5 fl. oz.	0	0	0	97	0	0
Whiskey	1.5 fl. oz.	0	0	0	105	0	0
Whiskey sour	3 fl. oz.	14	0	14	158	0	0

Food	Serving size	Carbohy-drates	Fiber	Net Carbs	Calories	Protein	Fat
FRUIT AND VEGETABLE JUICES AND BEVERAGES							
Apple juice, bottled	8 fl. oz.	29	0	29	117	0	0
Apple juice, from frozen concentrate	8 fl. oz.	28	0	28	112	0	0
Apricot nectar	8 fl. oz.	36	2	34	141	1	0
Capri Sun juice drink	8 fl. oz.	32	0	32	122	0	0
Carrot juice	8 fl. oz.	22	2	20	94	2	0
Cherry juice	8 fl. oz.	33	0	33	140	1	0
Clamato, Mott's	8 fl. oz.	24	0	24	110	1	0
Cranapple drink, Ocean Spray	8 fl. oz.	43	0	43	173	0	0
Cranberry juice cocktail	8 fl. oz.	37	0	37	144	0	0
Crangrape drink, Ocean Spray	8 fl. oz.	34	0	34	147	0	0
Crystal Lite mix, all flavors	8 fl. oz.	0	0	0	5	0	0
Fruit punch drink	8 fl. oz.	29	0	29	114	0	0
Grape juice, bottled	8 fl. oz.	38	0	38	154	1	0
Grape juice, from frozen concentrate	8 fl. oz.	32	0	32	128	0	0
Grapefruit juice, canned	8 fl. oz.	22	0	22	94	1	0
Grapefruit juice, fresh	8 fl. oz.	23	0	23	96	1	0

Food	Serving size	Carbohy-drates	Fiber	Net Carbs	Calories	Protein	Fat
Grapefruit juice, from frozen concentrate	8 fl. oz.	24	0	24	101	1	0
Grapefruit juice beverage, Carb Countdown	8 fl. oz.	5	0	5	25	0	0
Hawaiian Punch	8 fl. oz.	30	0	30	120	0	0
Hawaiian Punch, no sugar added	8 fl. oz.	4	0	4	15	0	0
Kool Aid mix, all flavors	8 fl. oz.	25	0	25	100	0	0
Kool Aid mix, sugar-free	8 fl. oz.	0	0	0	5	0	0
Lemonade, from frozen concentrate	8 fl. oz.	25	0	25	96	0	0
Lemonade, from powder mix	8 fl. oz.	27	0	27	103	0	0
Lemonade, from sugar-free powder mix	8 fl. oz.	0	0	0	5	0	0
Lemonade beverage, Carb Countdown	8 fl. oz.	4	0	4	20	0	0
Lemon juice	1 T	0	0	0	4	0	0
Lemon juice	8 fl. oz.	21	0	21	61	0	0
Lime juice	1 T	1	0	1	4	0	0
Lime juice	8 fl. oz.	22	0	22	66	0	0
Orange grapefruit juice	8 fl. oz.	25	0	25	106	0	0
Orange juice beverage, Carb Countdown	8 fl. oz.	5	0	5	25	0	0

Food	Serving size	Carbohy-drates	Fiber	Net Carbs	Calories	Protein	Fat
Orange juice, fresh	8 fl. oz.	26	0	26	112	2	0
Orange juice, from frozen concentrate	8 fl. oz.	27	0	27	112	2	0
Orange juice, refrigerated	8 fl. oz.	26	0	26	110	2	0
Orange juice, Light 'n Healthy, Tropicana	8 fl. oz.	13	0	13	50	0	0
Papaya nectar	8 fl. oz.	36	2	34	143	0	0
Peach nectar	8 fl. oz.	35	2	33	134	1	0
Pear nectar	8 fl. oz.	39	2	37	150	0	0
Pineapple grapefruit juice	8 fl. oz.	24	0	24	100	0	0
Pineapple juice	8 fl. oz.	34	0	34	140	1	0
Pineapple orange juice beverage, Carb Countdown	8 fl. oz.	5	0	5	25	0	0
Pineapple orange banana juice beverage, Carb Countdown	8 fl. oz.	5	0	5	25	0	0
Prune juice	8 fl. oz.	45	3	42	182	1	0
Sunny Delight Citrus Punch	8 fl. oz.	32	0	32	125	0	0
Tang	8 fl. oz.	29	0	29	115	0	0

Food	Serving size	Carbohydrates	Fiber	Net Carbs	Calories	Protein	Fat
Tang, sugar-free	8 fl. oz.	0	0	0	5	0	0
Tomato juice	8 fl. oz.	10	1	9	41	2	0
V-8 juice cocktail	8 fl. oz.	10	2	8	46	1	0

SPORT AND ENERGY BEVERAGES

Food	Serving size	Carbohydrates	Fiber	Net Carbs	Calories	Protein	Fat
AMP	8.4 fl. oz.	31	0	31	120	0	0
Fruit₂O	8 fl. oz.	0	0	0	0	0	0
Gatorade (all flavors)	12 fl. oz.	78	0	78	310	0	0
KMX	8 fl. oz.	31	0	31	118	0	0
PowerAde (all flavors)	8 fl. oz.	19	0	19	72	0	0
Propel Fitness Water (all flavors)	8 fl. oz.	3	0	3	10	0	0
Red Bull Energy Drink	8.3 fl. oz.	28	0	28	115	0	0
Red Bull Energy Drink, sugar-free	8.3 fl. oz.	3	0	3	15	0	0
Sobe Adrenaline Rush	8.3 fl. oz.	37	0	37	140	0	0

TEA, TEA BEVERAGES, AND HERBAL TEAS

Food	Serving size	Carbohy-drates	Fiber	Net Carbs	Calories	Protein	Fat
Chamomile tea	8 fl. oz.	0	0	0	2	0	0
Constant Comment brewed tea	8 fl. oz.	0	0	0	0	0	0
Iced tea, powder, artificial sweetener	8 fl. oz.	0	0	0	0	0	0
Iced tea, powder, sweetened	8 fl. oz.	19	0	19	80	0	0
Iced tea, powder, unsweetened	8 fl. oz.	0	0	0	2	0	0
Peppermint tea	8 fl. oz.	0	0	0	0	0	0
Tazo Chai Crème Frappucino	16 fl. oz.	72	0	72	380	13	5
Tazo Chai tea latte	16 fl. oz.	50	0	50	290	8	7
Tazo iced tea	16 fl. oz.	21	0	21	80	0	0
Tazo tea lemonade	16 fl. oz.	30	0	30	120	0	0
Tea, brewed, black	8 fl. oz.	1	0	1	2	0	0
Tea, brewed, green	8 fl. oz.	0	0	0	0	0	0

Food	Serving size	Carbohy-drates	Fiber	Net Carbs	Calories	Protein	Fat
WINE AND WINE BEVERAGES							
Port wine	6 fl. oz.	15	0	15	255	0	0
Sangria, Boone's Farm	12 fl. oz.	23	0	23	255	0	0
Sherry, cream	6 fl. oz.	15	0	15	255	0	0
Sherry, dry	6 fl. oz.	1.5	0	1.5	195	0	0
Wine cooler, Bartles & Jaymes	12 fl. oz.	30	0	30	210	0	0
Wine, red	3.5 fl. oz	2	0	2	74	0	0
Wine, rosé	3.5 fl. oz.	1	0	1	73	0	0
Wine spritzer	6 fl. oz.	3	0	3	70	0	0
Wine, white	3.5 fl. oz.	1	0	1	70	0	0

BREADS, MUFFINS, AND ROLLS

Here's where following the low-carb approach gets hard: cutting back on bread. For most people it's a big change, but most also find they can stick with it, especially as the pounds start to come off. As you lose weight and make the other lifestyle changes that are part of low-carbing, you can slowly introduce a bit more bread—preferably whole-grain bread—back into your diet. You can have a bit more if you use reduced-carb products.

TIP: Instead of a whole bagel, have just a half.

TIP: Get the most nutrition for your carbs by choosing whole-grain breads.

TIP: Ask for your burger on a plate, not a bun.

TIP: Be aware of portion size and carb counts when eating bread.

Food	Serving size	Carbohy-drates	Fiber	Net Carbs	Calories	Protein	Fat
Bagel, plain	1 bagel	56	2	54	289	11	2
Bagel, plain, Dunkin' Donuts	1 bagel	62	2	60	320	12	3
Bagel, cinnamon raisin	1 bagel	72	3	69	359	13	2
Bagel, cinnamon raisin, Dunkin' Donuts	1 bagel	65	3	62	330	10	3
Bagel, egg	1 bagel	56	2	54	292	11	2
Bagel, onion, Dunkin' Donuts	1 bagel	61	3	58	320	12	4
Biscuit, buttermilk, refrigerated dough, Pillsbury	1 biscuit	30	0	30	154	5	1
Biscuit, plain	1 biscuit	27	1	26	212	4	10
Biscuit, plain, refrigerated dough, Hungry Jack	1 biscuit	14	0	14	100	2	5
Biscuit, plain, refrigerated dough, Pillsbury	1 biscuit	29	0	29	150	4	2
Bread, banana	1 slice	33	1	32	196	3	6
Bread, Boston brown	1 slice	20	2	18	88	2	1
Bread, Bran'nola	1 slice	18	2	16	90	4	2
Bread, cracked wheat	1 slice	12	1	11	65	2	1
Bread, Crunchy Grains, Pepperidge Farm	1 slice	15	3	12	90	4	2

Food	Serving size	Carbohy-drates	Fiber	Net Carbs	Calories	Protein	Fat
Bread, French	1 slice	29	0	29	154	6	2
Bread, German dark wheat, Pepperidge Farm	1 slice	15	3	12	90	4	1
Bread, Health Nut, Arnold	1 slice	21	2	19	120	5	2
Bread, Healthy Multi-Grain, Arnold	1 slice	18	2	16	90	4	2
Bread, Hearty Bran, Pepperidge Farm	1 slice	15	3	12	90	4	2
Bread, Honey Oat, Pepperidge Farm	1 slice	15	2	13	90	4	2
Bread, Honey Wheat, Healthy Choice	1 slice	12	2	10	60	3	0
Bread, Irish soda	1 slice	16	1	15	82	2	1
Bread, Italian	1 slice	15	1	14	81	3	1
Bread, multigrain	1 slice	12	2	10	65	3	1
Bread, Multi Grain, Pepperidge Farm	1 slice	15	3	12	90	4	2
Bread, 9 Grain, Arnold	1 slice	18	3	15	100	4	2
Bread, 9 Grain, Pepperidge Farm	1 slice	15	3	12	90	4	1
Bread, oat bran	1 slice	12	1	11	71	3	1
Bread, Oat Bran, Arnold	1 slice	17	2	15	100	4	2
Bread, Oat Bran, Pepperidge Farm	1 slice	15	2	13	94	2	1

Food	Serving size	Carbohydrates	Fiber	Net Carbs	Calories	Protein	Fat
Bread, potato	1 slice	18	1	17	100	3	2
Bread, raisin	1 slice	14	1	13	71	2	1
Bread, Roman Meal	1 slice	13	1	12	69	3	1
Bread, rye	1 slice	16	2	14	83	3	1
Bread, sourdough	1 slice	33	2	31	175	6	2
Bread, wheat	1 slice	12	1	11	65	2	1
Bread, white	1 slice	12	1	11	67	2	1
Bread, white, Arnold	1 slice	19	0	19	110	3	2
Bread, whole wheat	1 slice	13	2	11	69	3	1
Bread, 100% whole wheat, Arnold	1 slice	18	3	15	90	4	1
Bread, Whole Wheat, Pepperidge Farm	1 slice	16	2	14	90	4	1
Bread crumbs	1 cup	78	3	75	427	14	6
Breadsticks, plain	1 stick	7	0	7	41	1	1
Cornbread	1 slice	29	0	29	18	4	6
Crescent roll	1 roll	11	0	11	110	2	6
Croissant	1 large	26	2	24	231	5	12
Croutons	1 cup	22	2	20	122	4	2

Food	Serving size	Carbohy-drates	Fiber	Net Carbs	Calories	Protein	Fat
Date nut loaf	1 slice	16	2	14	80	1	2
Dinner roll	1 roll	14	1	13	85	2	2
English muffin	1 muffin	26	0	26	132	5	1
English muffin, raisin cinnamon	1 muffin	28	2	26	139	4	2
English muffin, whole wheat	1 muffin	27	4	23	134	6	1
French roll	1 roll	19	1	18	105	3	2
Hamburger bun	1 bun	22	1	21	123	4	2
Hotdog roll	1 roll	22	1	21	123	4	2
Kaiser roll	1 roll	30	1	29	167	6	3
Muffin, blueberry	1 muffin	23	0	23	162	4	6
Muffin, bran	1 muffin	19	3	16	106	2	3
Muffin, corn	1 muffin	71	5	66	424	8	12
Muffin, oat bran	1 muffin	67	6	61	375	10	10
Pita, white	1 pita	33	1	32	165	6	1
Pita, whole wheat	1 pita	35	5	30	170	6	2
Pumpernickel	1 slice	12	2	10	65	2	1
Pumpernickel, Arnold	1 slice	16	1	15	80	2	1

Food	Serving size	Carbohy- drates	Fiber	Net Carbs	Calories	Protein	Fat
Taco shell	1 shell	7	0	7	50	2	1
Tortilla, corn	1 tortilla	11	1	10	53	1	1
Tortilla, flour	1 tortilla	26	2	24	150	4	3
Tostada shell	1 shell	7	0	7	50	1	2
Wrap, white, Sahara	1 wrap	29	1	28	170	5	5
Wrap, whole wheat, Sahara	1 wrap	27	4	23	170	5	5

REDUCED-CARB PRODUCTS

Food	Serving size	Carbohy- drates	Fiber	Net Carbs	Calories	Protein	Fat
Bagel, cinnamon raisin, Atkins	1 bagel	20	11	9	200	20	4
Bagel, onion, Atkins	1 bagel	19	11	8	190	19	4.5
Bagel, plain, Atkins	1 bagel	18	11	7	190	20	4.5
Bagel, reduced carb, Dunkin' Donuts	1 bagel	45	14	31	380	25	12
Bread, 7 Grain, Carb Style, Pepperidge Farm	1 slice	8	3	5	60	5	2
Bread, white, Carb Style, Pepperidge Farm	1 slice	8	3	5	60	5	1
Bread, 100% Whole Wheat, Carb Style, Pepperidge Farm	1 slice	8	3	5	60	5	2

Food	Serving size	Carbohy-drates	Fiber	Net Carbs	Calories	Protein	Fat
Dinner roll, Carb Monitor	1 roll	11	4	7	70	6	2
Muffin, banana nut, Atkins	1 muffin	20	9	11	190	5	13
Muffin, blueberry, Atkins	1 muffin	20	8	12	130	4	7
Pita, Atkins	1 pita	17	11	6	80	10	2
Tortilla, garlic and herb, La Tortilla Factory	1 tortilla	11	8	3	50	5	2
Tortilla, green onion, La Tortilla Factory	1 tortilla	11	8	3	50	5	2
Tortilla, large original, La Tortilla Factory	1 tortilla	19	14	5	80	8	3
Tortilla, original, La Tortilla Factory	1 tortilla	11	8	3	50	5	2

Food	Serving size	Carbohydrates	Fiber	Sugar Alcohol	Net Carbs	Calories	Protein	Fat
REDUCED-CARB BAKE MIXES								
Bake mix, Atkins	⅛ cup	8	5	0	3	80	13	0.5
Bake mix, Carb Solutions	⅛ cup	6	3	0	3	110	18	2
Banana nut muffin, Carb Fit	3 T mix prepared	10	4	0	6	100	8	2.5
Batter mix, Atkins	2 T mix prepared	5	4	0	1	30	3	0
Biscuit mix, Atkins	1 biscuit	4	3	0	1	25	4	0
Blueberry muffin, Carb Fit	3 T mix prepared	12	4	0	6	100	7	1.5
Blueberry muffin, Carb Solutions	2 T mix prepared	9	2	0	7	130	8	0
Bun mix, Atkins	1 bun	4	3	0	1	23	4	0
Caraway rye bread, Atkins	1 slice	8	5	0	3	70	12	0
Carb Simple Country White Bread, Krusteaz	½ cup mix prepared	16	7	0	9	140	11	3

Food	Serving size	Carbohy-drates	Fiber	Sugar Alcohol	Net Carbs	Calories	Protein	Fat
Carb Simple wild blueberry muffin mix, Krusteaz	½ cup mix prepared	20	4	7	9	170	7	5
Corn muffin, Carb Solutions	2 T mix prepared	9	2	0	7	130	8	0
Country white bread, Atkins	¼ cup mix prepared	8	5	0	3	70	12	0
Sourdough bread, Atkins	1 slice	8	5	0	3	70	12	0
Wild blueberry muffin mix, Betty Crocker Carb Monitor	2 T mix prepared	27	6	5	16	160	2	1.5

BREAKFAST CEREALS

Whether you eat them for breakfast, as a snack, or even for dinner, breakfast cereals are a favorite food—and everyone has a favorite brand. Unsweetened whole-grain cereals are relatively low in net carbs and can be a part of your diet, as long as you watch the portions and stay aware of the net carbs. To keep the carb count down, try adding a reduced-carb milk beverage instead of milk.

TIP: Choose high-fiber cereals to limit net carbs.

TIP: Old-fashioned oats have the most fiber.

TIP: Use small amounts of fresh fruit instead of sugar on your cereal.

COLD CEREALS (portions are dry without milk)

Food	Serving size	Carbohy-drates	Fiber	Net Carbs	Calories	Protein	Fat
All-Bran	1 cup	23	10	13	81	4	1
Alpha-Bits	1 cup	27	1	26	130	3	1
Apple Jacks	1 cup	27	1	26	117	1	1
Apple Cinnamon Squares	¾ cup	44	5	39	182	4	1
Banana Nut Crunch	1 cup	43	4	39	250	5	6
Basic 4	1 cup	42	3	39	202	4	3
Blueberry Morning	1¼ cups	43	2	41	211	4	3
Boo Berry	1 cup	27	0	27	118	1	1
Bran, 100%	⅓ cup	23	8	15	83	4	1
Bran Flakes	¾ cup	24	5	19	96	3	1
Cap'n Crunch	¾ cup	23	1	22	108	1	2
Cap'n Crunch Crunchberries	¾ cup	22	1	21	104	1	2
Cap'n Crunch Peanut Butter	¾ cup	21	1	20	112	2	3
Cheerios	1 cup	22	3	19	111	3	2
Cheerios, apple cinnamon	¾ cup	25	1	24	118	2	2
Cheerios, honey nut	1 cup	24	2	22	112	3	1

Food	Serving size	Carbohy-drates	Fiber	Net Carbs	Calories	Protein	Fat
Cheerios, frosted	1 cup	26	1	25	115	2	1
Cheerios multi-grain	1 cup	24	3	21	108	2	1
Chex, corn	1 cup	26	1	25	112	2	0
Chex, frosted mini	¾ cup	27	0	27	110	1	0
Chex, honey nut	¾ cup	26	0	26	114	2	1
Chex, multi-bran	1 cup	41	6	35	166	3	1
Chex, rice	1¼ cups	27	0	27	117	2	0
Chex, wheat	1 cup	24	3	21	104	3	1
Cinnamon Grahams	¾ cup	26	1	25	113	2	1
Cinnamon Oatmeal Squares	1 cup	48	5	43	227	6	3
Cinnamon Toast Crunch	¾ cup	24	1	23	127	2	3
Cocoa Blasts	1 cup	29	1	28	130	1	1
Cocoa Krispies	¾ cup	27	1	26	118	1	1
Cocoa Pebbles	¾ cup	25	1	24	115	1	1
Cocoa Puffs	1 cup	26	1	25	117	1	1
Cookie Crisp	1 cup	26	1	25	117	1	1
Corn flakes, Kellogg's	1 cup	24	1	23	102	2	0

Food	Serving size	Carbohy-drates	Fiber	Net Carbs	Calories	Protein	Fat
Corn Pops	1 cup	28	0	28	118	1	0
Count Chocula	1 cup	26	0	26	119	1	1
Crispix	1 cup	25	0	25	109	2	0
Crispy rice	1 cup	25	0	25	111	2	0
Crispy Wheaties 'n' Raisins	1 cup	45	5	40	183	4	1
Crunchy Bran	¾ cup	23	5	18	90	2	1
CW Post	¼ cup	21	4	17	122	2	4
CW Post with raisins	¼ cup	20	5	15	121	2	4
Fiber One	½ cup	24	14	10	59	2	1
Frankenberry	1 cup	27	0	27	118	1	1
Froot Loops	1 cup	26	1	25	118	1	1
Frosted Flakes	¾ cup	28	1	27	114	1	0
Frosted Krispies	¾ cup	27	0	27	114	1	0
Frosted Mini-Wheats	1 cup	45	6	39	189	6	1
Fruit & Fibre	1 cup	42	5	37	212	4	3
Fruity Pebbles	¾ cup	24	0	23	108	1	1
Golden Crisp	¾ cup	25	0	25	107	2	0

Food	Serving size	Carbohy-drates	Fiber	Net Carbs	Calories	Protein	Fat
Golden Grahams	¾ cup	25	1	24	112	2	1
Granola, fruit, Nature Valley	2 oz.	44	3	41	212	4	3
Granola, Post	⅔ cup	45	3	42	280	5	9
Granola, low-fat, Kellogg's	½ cup	39	3	36	186	4	3
Granola, Nature Valley	½ cup	18	3	15	126	3	5
Granola, oats and honey, Quaker	½ cup	31	3	28	219	5	9
Grape-Nut Flakes	¾ cup	24	3	21	106	3	1
Grape-Nuts	½ cup	47	5	42	208	6	1
Great Grains, crunch pecan	½ cup	38	4	34	216	5	6
Harmony	1¼ cups	44	2	42	200	5	1
Heartland Natural	1 cup	79	7	72	499	12	18
Honey Bunches of Oats	¾ cup	25	2	23	118	2	2
Honey Bunches of Oats, almonds	¾ cup	24	1	23	126	2	3
Honey Graham Oh!s	¾ cup	23	1	22	111	1	2
Honey Nut Clusters	1 cup	46	3	43	214	4	3
Honeycomb	1⅓ cups	26	1	25	115	2	1
Kashi GoLean	1 cup	30	10	20	140	13	1

Food	Serving size	Carbohy-drates	Fiber	Net Carbs	Calories	Protein	Fat
Kashi GoLean crunch	1 cup	36	8	28	190	9	3
Kashi Heart to Heart	¾ cup	25	5	20	110	4	1.5
Kashi Seven in the Morning	½ cup	47	7	40	210	7	1.5
Kellogg's Corn flakes	1 cup	24	1	23	101	2	0
King Vitaman	1½ cups	26	1	25	120	2	1
Kix	1⅓ cup	26	1	25	113	2	1
Life	¾ cup	25	2	23	120	3	1
Life, cinnamon	¾ cup	26	2	24	120	3	1
Lucky Charms	1 cup	25	2	23	114	2	1
Muesli, Familia	½ cup	45	4	41	210	6	3
Muesli, Sunbelt	2 oz.	42	4	38	206	5	2
Muselix, raisin almond with dates	2 oz.	40	4	36	196	5	3
Oat Bran Flakes, Common Sense	¾ cup	23	4	19	105	3	1
Oat Bran, Quaker	1¼ cups	43	6	37	212	7	3
Oatmeal Crisp, almond	1 cup	42	4	38	218	6	5
Oatmeal Crisp, apple	1 cup	45	4	41	207	5	2
Oatmeal Crisp, raisin	1 cup	45	4	41	204	5	2

Food	Serving size	Carbohy-drates	Fiber	Net Carbs	Calories	Protein	Fat
Oatmeal Squares	1 cup	44	4	40	212	6	2
Product 19	1 cup	25	1	24	109	2	0
Puffed rice	1 cup	13	0	13	56	1	0
Puffed wheat	1 cup	10	0	10	44	2	0
Quaker 100% Natural granola	½ cup	37	3	34	210	5	6
Raisin bran, Kellogg's	1 cup	45	7	38	188	5	2
Raisin bran, Post	1 cup	46	8	38	187	5	1
Raisin Nut Bran	1 cup	42	5	37	209	5	4
Rice Krispies	1¼ cups	29	0	29	128	2	0
Shredded Wheat, Post	2 biscuits	38	5	33	156	5	0
Smacks, Kellogg's	¾ cup	24	1	23	104	2	0
Smart Start	1 cup	43	2	41	182	3	1
Special K	1 cup	22	1	21	117	7	0
Total	¾ cup	23	2	21	97	2	1
Trix	1 cup	27	1	26	117	1	1
Wheaties	1 cup	24	3	21	107	3	1

Food	Serving size	Carbohydrates	Fiber	Net Carbs	Calories	Protein	Fat
REDUCED-CARB PRODUCTS							
Banana Nut Harvest, Atkins	½ cup	11	6	5	100	12	3
Blueberry Bounty with Almonds, Atkins	½ cup	10	6	4	100	13	2
CarbWell Cinnamon Crunch	1 oz.	14	5	9	118	11	2
CarbWell Golden Crunch	1 oz.	14	5	9	118	11	1
Crunchy Almond Crisp, Atkins	½ cup	8	5	3	100	15	2
Frosted flakes, honey nut, Keto	¾ cup	9	2	7	110	17	1
Granola, apple cinnamon, MiniCarb	½ cup	29	25	4	285	8	15
Triple Berry, Atkins	½ cup	10	6	4	90	14	2
HOT CEREALS (all portions are cooked)							
Corn grits	1 cup	32	1	31	145	3	0
Cream of rice	1 cup	28	0	28	127	2	0
Cream of wheat	1 cup	28	2	26	133	4	0
Farina	1 cup	25	3	22	117	3	0
Hominy grits	1 cup	32	1	31	324	3	0

Food	Serving size	Carbohy-drates	Fiber	Net Carbs	Calories	Protein	Fat
Kashi Heart to Heart instant oatmeal	1 packet	33	5	28	160	4	2
Kashi instant oatmeal, golden brown maple	1 packet	33	5	28	160	4	2
Maltex	½ cup	37	5	32	170	5	0
Maypo	1 cup	32	6	26	170	6	2
Oat bran	1 cup	18	4	14	101	5	2
Oatmeal, instant	1 cup	24	4	20	138	6	2
Oatmeal, instant, apple cinnamon	1 packet	27	3	24	125	3	1.5
Oatmeal, instant, bran and raisins	1 packet	30	6	24	158	5	2
Oatmeal, instant, cinnamon spice	1 packet	35	3	32	177	5	2
Oatmeal, instant, raisin spice	1 packet	32	2	30	161	4	2
Oatmeal, regular/quick	1 cup	25	4	21	145	6	2
Wheatena	1 cup	29	7	22	136	5	1

REDUCED-CARB PRODUCTS

Food	Serving size	Carbohy-drates	Fiber	Net Carbs	Calories	Protein	Fat
Apple Cinnamon, Atkins	½ cup	8	5	3	70	12	1
Cinnamon and Spice, Atkins	½ cup	8	5	3	90	12	1
Country Spice, Carbsense	½ cup	15	12	3	170	12	7

Food	Serving size	Carbohy-drates	Fiber	Net Carbs	Calories	Protein	Fat
Harvest Blend, Carb Fit	¼ cup	12	8	4	180	17	7
Natural, Atkins	½ cup	8	5	3	90	12	1
Peaches and Cream, Atkins	½ cup	8	5	3	90	12	1
Sweet Maple, Atkins	½ cup	8	5	3	90	12	1

BREAKFAST PASTRIES: PANCAKES, WAFFLES, TOASTER PASTRIES

A lot of traditional breakfast foods such as pancakes are unfortunately high in carbs. If you're watching your carb intake, these foods may have to become only occasional treats—Sunday brunch, for instance. Limit the carbs by choosing low-carb toppings such as fresh berries or sugar-free syrup.

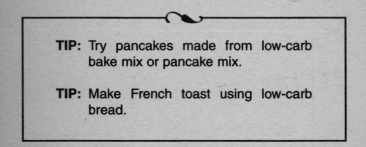

TIP: Try pancakes made from low-carb bake mix or pancake mix.

TIP: Make French toast using low-carb bread.

Food	Serving size	Carbohy-drates	Fiber	Net Carbs	Calories	Protein	Fat
French toast, frozen	1 piece	19	0	19	126	4	4
French toast, homemade	1 piece	16	0	16	151	5	7
Pancake, blueberry, homemade	1 pancake	11	2	9	84	2	4
Pancake, blueberry, microwave	1 pancake	15	1	14	77	2	2
Pancake, buckwheat, mix	1 pancake	8	0	8	62	2	2
Pancake, buttermilk, homemade	1 pancake	11	0	10	86	3	4
Pancake, buttermilk, Eggo	3 pancakes	44	1	43	270	7	8
Pancake, buttermilk, microwave	1 pancake	15	0	15	80	2	2
Pancake, plain, homemade	1 pancake	11	0	11	86	2	4
Pancake, plain, microwave	1 pancake	16	0	16	86	2	1
Pancake, plain, mix	1 pancake	14	0	14	74	2	1
Pancake, plain, mix, Shake 'n Pour, Bisquick	1 pancake	13	0	13	67	2	1
Toaster muffin, blueberry	1 muffin	15	1	14	88	1	3
Toaster muffin, corn	1 muffin	16	2	14	97	2	3
Toaster muffin, wheat bran	1 muffin	15	3	12	83	1	3
Toaster pastry, apple cinnamon, Pop-Tart	1 pastry	37	1	36	210	2	6
Toaster pastry, blueberry, Pop-Tart	1 pastry	36	1	35	197	2	5

Food	Serving size	Carbohy-drates	Fiber	Net Carbs	Calories	Protein	Fat
Toaster pastry, chocolate chip, Pop-Tart	1 pastry	35	1	34	215	3	7
Toaster pastry, strawberry, Pop-Tart	1 pastry	37	1	36	201	2	5
Toast-R-Cakes	1 cake	17	1	16	103	2	4
Waffle, banana bread, Eggo	1 waffle	32	2	30	212	5	7
Waffle, blueberry, Eggo	1 waffle	15	1	14	73	2	1
Waffle, blueberry, homemade	1 waffle	30	2	28	186	6	5
Waffle, buttermilk, homemade	1 waffle	25	1	24	217	6	10
Waffle, buttermilk, Eggo	1 waffle	16	2	14	95	3	4
Waffle, buttermilk, Hungry Man	1 waffle	15	1	14	95	4	6
Waffle, homestyle, Eggo	1 waffle	15	1	14	100	3	4
Waffle, oat, Eggo	1 waffle	13	1	12	69	2	1
Waffle, plain, homemade	1 waffle	25	0	25	218	6	10
Waffle, plain, mix	1 waffle	23	0	23	207	6	10
Waffle, plain, Hungry Jack	1 waffle	17	1	16	65	2	1
Waffle, plain, Nutri-Grain, Eggo	1 waffle	14	1	13	71	2	1
Waffle, plain, Aunt Jemima	1 waffle	15	0	15	97	3	3

Food	Serving size	Carbohy-drates	Fiber	Net Carbs	Calories	Protein	Fat
REDUCED-CARB PRODUCTS							
Pancake, buttermilk, mix, CarbSense	1 pancake	2	1	1	106	10	5
Pancake, plain, mix, Atkins	1 pancake	4	2	2	35	4	0
Pancake, plain, mix, Carbolite	1 pancake	10	6	5	100	21	0
Pancake, plain, mix, Simple Chef, Carb Solutions	1 pancake	5	2	3	80	8	0
Waffle, plain, Atkins	1 waffle	9	2	7	130	6	9

CANDY

Your sweet tooth is in for a surprise when you start low carbing—there are now a lot of delicious low-carb candies! To provide sweetness without carb grams, the candy manufacturers replace sugar and high-fructose corn syrup with sugar alcohols such as maltitol, then deduct the sugar alcohols from the total carbohydrate grams to get a low net carb number. There's some controversy about how much of the sugar alcohols you absorb, so be aware of both the total and net carb counts. In addition, some people are sensitive to sugar alcohols and may have digestive upsets if they eat more than a small amount.

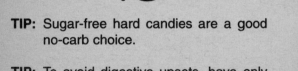

TIP: Sugar-free hard candies are a good no-carb choice.

TIP: To avoid digestive upsets, have only small amounts of sugar-free candy.

Food	Serving size	Carbohy-drates	Fiber	Net Carbs	Calories	Protein	Fat
After Eight Mints	5 mints	32	1	31	147	1	6
Almond Joy	1 bar	11	1	10	91	1	5
Almond Joy Bites	18 pieces	23	2	21	218	2	14
Baby Ruth	1 bar	39	2	37	289	5	13
Butterfinger	1 bar	40	2	38	293	8	11
Butterscotch	5 pieces	26	0	26	111	0	1
Caramels	10 pieces	55	1	54	271	4	6
Chocolate-coated almonds	12 pieces	19	2	17	234	5	6
Chocolate-coated peanuts	10 pieces	20	2	18	208	5	13
Chocolate-coated raisins	¼ cup	31	2	29	176	2	7
Chocolate, dark	1 oz.	17	0	17	138	1	9
Chunky	1 piece	23	2	21	198	4	12
Crunch	1 bar	29	0	29	230	3	12
Fifth Avenue	1 bar	35	2	33	270	5	13
Fudge	1 oz.	26	1	25	140	1	4
Goobers	1 package	19	2	17	200	5	13
Good & Plenty	snack box	14	0	14	60	0	0

Food	Serving size	Carbohy-drates	Fiber	Net Carbs	Calories	Protein	Fat
Gum drops	10 pieces	36	0	36	139	0	0
Gummy bears	10 pieces	22	0	22	85	0	0
Heath Bar	1 bar	6	0	6	50	0	3
Jelly beans	1 oz.	26	0	26	103	0	0
Jolly Rancher	2 pieces	17	0	17	70	0	0
Kisses	1 piece	3	0	3	25	0	0
Kit Kat Wafer	1 bar	50	1	49	403	5	21
Krackel	1 bar	36	1	35	287	4	9
M&M's Peanut	25 pieces	30	2	28	253	5	13
M&M's Plain	70 pieces	34	1	33	236	2	10
Marshmallow	1 piece	6	0	6	23	0	0
Milk chocolate	1.5 oz	26	2	24	226	3	14
Milk chocolate chips	1 cup	100	6	94	862	12	52
Milk Duds	7 pieces	15	0	15	90	0	4
Milky Way	1 bar	43	1	42	254	3	10
Mint wafer crisp bars	2 bars	15	3	4	120	4	9
Mounds	1 bar	31	2	29	258	2	14

Food	Serving size	Carbohy-drates	Fiber	Net Carbs	Calories	Protein	Fat
Mr. Goodbar	1 bar	27	2	25	264	5	16
Oh Henry!	1 bar	37	2	35	246	6	10
Payday	1 bar	10	0	10	90	2	5
Peanut brittle	1 oz.	20	1	19	134	2	5
Raisinets	1 package	32	0	32	185	2	7
Reese's Peanut Butter Cups	2 pieces	25	2	23	232	5	14
Reese's Pieces	58 pieces	28	1	27	229	6	11
Skittles Candies	54 pieces	52	0	54	231	0	3
Skor Toffee Bar	1 bar	24	0	24	209	1	13
Snickers	1 bar	34	1	33	273	5	14
Starburst Fruit Chews	6 pieces	50	0	50	234	0	5
Symphony	1 bar	24	1	23	223	4	13
Three Musketeers	1 bar	46	1	45	250	2	8
Twix Cookie Bar	2 bars	38	1	37	289	3	14
Twizzlers, strawberry	2.5 oz.	57	0	57	249	2	2
Whoppers malted milk balls	10 pieces	15	0	15	90	0	4
York Peppermint Patty	1 patty	35	1	34	165	1	3
Zero	1 bar	12	0	12	70	1	3

Food	Serving size	Carbohy-drates	Fiber	Sugar Alcohol	Net Carbs	Calories	Protein	Fat
REDUCED-CARB PRODUCTS								
Chocolate, Carb Solutions	1 bar	17	0	14	3	140	3	10
Chocolate caramel, Carb Solutions	1 bar	18	0	15	3	130	2	8
Chocolate crisp, Carb Solutions	1 bar	16	0	13	3	140	5	9
Chocolate mints, Calorie Smart, Russell Stover	1 piece	8	0	7	1	5	2	4
Chocolate wafer crisp bars, Atkins	2 bars	15	3	8	4	120	4	9
Coconut almond clusters, Carb Solutions	3 clusters	19	0	17	2	120	2	8
Minicarb milk chocolate bars, Carbsense	1 bar	14	13	0	1	170	4	11
Mint Patties, Russell Stover Low Carb	2 pieces	19	0	18	1	130	2	7
Peanut butter cups, Carb Solutions	3 cups	17	0	15	2	140	3	10
Peanut butter wafer crisp bars, Atkins	2 bars	14	3	7	4	120	4	9
Pecan Delights, Russell Stover Low Carb	2 pieces	16	2	13	1	130	2	10
Toffee Squares, Russell Stover Low Carb	2 pieces	16	0	15	1	110	2	7
Vanilla wafer crisp bars, Atkins	2 bars	15	3	8	4	120	4	9

CANNED AND PACKAGED ENTREES

This category includes convenient prepared foods sold in cans or packaged portions. Today these foods are often available in single-serve portions that can be easily prepared in the microwave. It's important to balance the convenience of these foods against their carbohydrate content. It's also important to be aware of portion size. In many cases, the single serving is large, or the container actually has two portions. It's all too easy to eat the whole thing and get more carbs and calories than you realize.

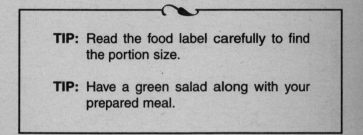

TIP: Read the food label carefully to find the portion size.

TIP: Have a green salad along with your prepared meal.

Food	Serving size	Carbohy-drates	Fiber	Net Carbs	Calories	Protein	Fat
Baked beans with franks	1 cup	40	18	22	368	18	17
Baked beans with pork	1 cup	51	14	37	268	13	4
Beefaroni, Chef Boyardee	1 serving	31	3	28	184	8	3
Beef ravioli, tomato sauce, Chef Boyardee	1 cup	37	4	33	229	8	5
Beef stew, Dinty Moore	1 cup	16	3	13	222	22	13
Beef stew, Hormel	1 container	15	0	15	190	10	10
Beef stew, Trader Joe's	1 cup	21	3	18	239	14	11
Beef Stroganoff, Betty Crocker	1 serving	34	0	34	225	11	5
Chicken and buttermilk biscuits, Betty Crocker	1 serving	41	2	39	321	10	13
Chicken and dumplings, Dinty Moore	1 cup	24	2	23	194	11	6
Chicken fettuccine alfredo, Betty Crocker	1 serving	38	2	36	307	14	11
Chicken Helper, cheddar and broccoli	1 cup	28	0	28	310	27	9
Chicken Helper, fettuccini alfredo	1 cup	28	1	27	290	26	8
Chicken Helper, southwestern chicken	1 cup	27	1	26	240	23	5
Chili con carne, no beans	1 serving	25	8	17	255	20	8
Chili con carne, no beans, Hormel	1 cup	18	3	15	194	17	7

Food	Serving size	Carbohy-drates	Fiber	Net Carbs	Calories	Protein	Fat
Chili con carne, beans	1 cup	31	11	20	287	15	14
Chili con carne, beans, Hormel	1 cup	34	8	26	240	17	4
Chili con carne, beans, Old El Paso	1 cup	22	10	12	249	18	10
Chili Magic, traditional, Bush's	1 cup	38	10	28	220	10	2
Chili, vegetarian, Hormel	1 cup	38	10	28	205	12	1
Corned beef hash, Armour	1 cup	12	2	10	498	24	39
Corned beef hash, Hormel	1 cup	22	3	19	387	21	24
Ham and au gratin potatoes, Betty Crocker	1 serving	37	2	35	297	8	13
Hamburger Helper, cheddar and broccoli	1 cup	31	0	31	270	14	11
Hamburger Helper, chili mac	1 cup	30	1	29	300	20	12
Hamburger Helper, Stroganoff	1 cup	30	0	30	320	21	13
Hamburger Helper, zesty Italian	1 cup	32	2	30	300	20	10
Macaroni and cheese	1 serving	29	3	26	199	8	6
Macaroni and cheese, Kraft	1 serving	44	4	40	318	13	10
Noodles and sauce, Lipton	1 cup	42	2	40	307	6	12
Pasta and sauce, Lipton	1 cup	45	1	44	311	6	10
Pasta with franks	1 cup	30	2	28	262	9	12

Food	Serving size	Carbohy-drates	Fiber	Net Carbs	Calories	Protein	Fat
Pasta with meatballs	1 cup	31	7	24	260	11	10
Ravioli, beef, Buitoni	1 serving	48	2	46	342	15	10
Spaghetti Os, sliced franks	1 cup	27	5	22	234	9	5
Spaghetti Os, meatballs	1 cup	32	3	29	244	11	4
Spaghetti Os, original	1 cup	37	3	34	181	6	1
Tortellini, spinach and cheese, Buitoni	1 serving	49	3	46	328	15	8
Tortellini, three-cheese, Buitoni	1 serving	50	3	47	323	15	7
Tuna Helper, cheesy broccoli	1 cup	34	1	33	290	15	9
Tuna Helper, creamy pasta	1 cup	32	2	30	290	12	13
Tuna Helper, garden cheddar	1 cup	36	1	35	290	13	11
Tuna Helper, tetrazzini	1 cup	34	1	33	300	14	12
Tuna Helper, tuna melt	1 cup	34	0	34	300	12	13

CHEESE AND CHEESE PRODUCTS

Cheese is a mainstay of the low-carb lifestyle. The many varieties of cheese provide a lot of ways to add flavor and interest to vegetable dishes, casseroles, and salads. It's convenient, too—individually packaged cheese portions can easily go into a lunch bag or snack pack. Be aware, though, that cheese is high in calories. A standard portion is only an ounce—that's the amount in one slice of prewrapped processed cheese.

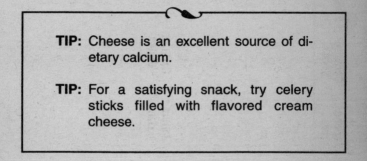

TIP: Cheese is an excellent source of dietary calcium.

TIP: For a satisfying snack, try celery sticks filled with flavored cream cheese.

Food	Serving size	Carbohy-drates	Fiber	Net Carbs	Calories	Protein	Fat
American cheese, processed	1 oz.	1	0	1	106	6	9
American cheese, processed, Kraft	1 oz.	1	0	1	110	5	9
American cheese food	1 oz.	2	0	2	93	6	7
American cheese food, Kraft	1 oz.	2	0	2	90	5	6
American cheese spread	1 oz.	3	0	3	82	5	6
Blue	1 oz.	1	0	1	100	6	8
Brick	1 oz.	1	0	1	105	7	8
Brie	1 oz.	0	0	0	95	6	8
Butterkäse	1 oz.	0	0	0	100	6	9
Camembert	1 oz.	0	0	0	85	6	7
Cheddar	1 oz.	0	0	0	114	7	9
Cheddar, horseradish	1 oz.	2	0	2	110	6	9
cheddar, low-fat	1 oz.	1	0	1	49	7	2
Cheddar, low-sodium	1 oz.	1	0	1	113	7	9
Cheese sauce, cheddar, Land O' Lakes	1 oz.	3	0	3	38	1	3
Cheese spread, Cheez Whiz	2 T	2	0	2	90	5	7
Cheese spread, Velveeta	1 oz.	3	0	3	80	5	6

Food	Serving size	Carbohy-drates	Fiber	Net Carbs	Calories	Protein	Fat
Cheshire	1 oz.	1	0	1	110	7	9
Colby	1 oz.	1	0	1	112	7	9
Cottage cheese, 1% fat	1 cup	6	0	6	164	28	2
Cottage cheese, 2% fat	1 cup	8	0	8	203	31	4
Cottage cheese, creamed	1 cup	6	0	6	217	26	10
Cottage cheese, dry curd	1 cup	3	0	3	123	25	1
Cream cheese	1 oz.	1	0	1	99	2	10
Cream cheese, fat-free	1 oz.	2	0	2	30	5	0
Cream cheese, whipped	3 T	1	0	1	110	2	11
Double Gloucester	1 oz.	0	0	0	110	7	10
Edam	1 oz.	0	0	0	101	7	8
Farmers	1 oz.	1	0	1	100	6	8
Feta	1 oz.	1	0	1	75	4	6
Fontina	1 oz.	0	0	0	110	7	9
Goat, soft	1 oz.	1	0	1	76	4	6
Gouda	1 oz.	2	0	2	101	5	8
Gruyere	1 oz.	0	0	0	117	9	9

Food	Serving size	Carbohy-drates	Fiber	Net Carbs	Calories	Protein	Fat
Havarti	1 oz.	0	0	0	120	6	11
Jalapeño jack	1 oz.	1	0	1	90	5	8
Monterey jack	1 oz.	0	0	0	106	7	9
Mozzarella, part skim	1 oz.	1	0	1	72	7	5
Mozzarella, string	1 oz.	1	0	1	80	7	6
Mozzarella, whole milk	1 oz.	1	0	1	80	6	6
Muenster	1 oz.	0	0	0	104	7	9
Neufchatel	1 oz.	1	0	1	74	3	7
Parmesan, grated	1 T	0	0	0	23	2	2
Provolone	1 oz.	0	0	0	100	7	8
Ricotta, part skim	½ cup	6	0	6	171	14	10
Ricotta, whole milk	½ cup	4	0	4	216	14	16
Romano, grated	1 oz.	1	0	1	110	9	8
Roquefort	1 oz.	1	0	1	105	6	9
Swiss	1 oz.	1	0	1	107	8	8
Swiss, Kraft	1 slice	1	0	1	70	4	5
Swiss cheese food	1 oz.	1	0	1	92	6	7
Swiss, processed	1 oz.	1	0	1	95	7	7

COLD CUTS

No matter what you call them—cold cuts, sandwich meats, deli meats, luncheon meats—they're all good choices when you're following the low-carb approach. These flavorful meats are precooked and store well in the fridge, making them very convenient for quick meals and snacks. Cold cuts come in many varieties, but check the labels carefully. Products such as bologna, olive loaf, and hot dogs may contain fillers that add carbs.

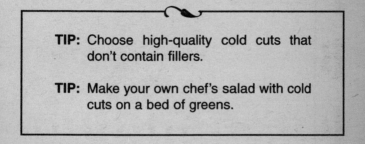

TIP: Choose high-quality cold cuts that don't contain fillers.

TIP: Make your own chef's salad with cold cuts on a bed of greens.

Food	Serving size	Carbohydrates	Fiber	Net Carbs	Calories	Protein	Fat
Beef sausage, smoked	1.5 oz.	1	0	1	134	6	12
Bologna, beef	1 oz.	0	0	0	87	3	8
Bologna, beef, Boar's Head	2 oz.	0	0	0	150	7	13
Bologna, beef, Oscar Mayer	1 oz.	1	0	1	88	3	8
Bologna, fat free, Oscar Mayer	1 oz.	2	0	2	22	4	0
Bologna, pork	1 oz.	0	0	0	69	4	6
Bologna, turkey	1 oz.	0	0	0	56	4	4
Bratwurst, Boar's Head	4 oz.	0	0	0	300	19	25
Bratwurst, pork	3 oz.	2	0	2	256	12	22
Bratwurst, veal	3 oz.	0	0	0	288	12	27
Capocollo, Boar's Head	1 oz.	0	0	0	80	7	5
Chicken breast, roasted, Boar's Head	2 oz.	0	0	0	60	13	1
Chicken breast, Buffalo, Boar's Head	2 oz.	0	0	0	60	13	1
Chicken roll, roasted	2 oz.	1	0	1	75	8	4
Chorizo	2 oz.	1	0	1	273	15	23
Corned beef, Boar's Head	2 oz.	0	0	0	80	12	4
Dutch loaf, Boar's Head	2 oz.	2	0	2	150	7	12

Food	Serving size	Carbohy-drates	Fiber	Net Carbs	Calories	Protein	Fat
Frankfurter, beef	1.5 oz.	2	0	2	141	5	13
Frankfurter, beef, Boar's Head	2 oz.	0	0	0	120	6	11
Frankfurter, fat-free, Oscar Mayer	1.8 oz.	3	0	3	39	7	0
Frankfurter, Oscar Mayer	2 oz.	2	0	2	185	6	17
Ham	1 oz.	1	0	1	51	5	3
Ham, Black Forest, Boar's Head	2 oz.	2	0	2	60	10	1
Ham, Boar's Head	2 oz.	2	0	2	60	9	1
Ham, cappy, Boar's Head	2 oz.	3	0	3	60	10	2
Ham, maple-glazed, Boar's Head	2 oz.	3	0	3	60	10	1
Ham, spiced	2 oz.	1	0	1	120	7	10
Ham, Virginia, Boar's Head	2 oz.	2	0	2	60	9	1
Knockwurst, beef, Boar's Head	4 oz.	1	0	1	310	15	27
Liverwurst	1 oz.	0	0	0	110	5	10
Liverwurst, smoked, Boar's Head	2 oz.	1	0	1	170	8	15
Luncheon loaf, spiced, Oscar Mayer	1 oz.	2	0	2	66	4	5
Mortadella	1 oz.	1	0	1	94	3	4
Mortadella, Boar's Head	2 oz.	0	0	0	160	9	14

Food	Serving size	Carbohy-drates	Fiber	Net Carbs	Calories	Protein	Fat
Olive loaf	1 oz.	3	0	3	66	3	5
Olive loaf, Boar's Head	2 oz.	0	0	0	130	6	12
Olive loaf, Oscar Mayer	1 oz.	2	0	2	74	3	6
Pastrami	1 oz.	1	0	1	98	5	8
Pastrami, Boar's Head	2 oz.	2	0	2	90	12	4
Pepperoni	1 oz.	1	0	1	135	6	12
Pepperoni, Boar's Head	1 oz.	1	0	1	130	5	12
Prosciutto, Boar's Head	1 oz.	0	0	0	60	8	3
Roast beef, Boar's Head	2 oz.	0	0	0	90	14	3
Salami, beef	1 oz.	0	0	0	88	5	8
Salami, beef, Boar's Head	2 oz.	0	0	0	120	10	9
Salami, Genoa, Boar's Head	2 oz.	1	0	1	180	12	14
Salami, Genoa, Oscar Mayer	1 oz.	0	0	0	105	6	9
Salami, hard, Boar's Head	2 oz.	0	0	0	110	6	9
Salami, hard, Oscar Mayer	1 oz.	0	0	0	99	7	8
Smoked sausage, beef, Oscar Mayer	1.5 oz.	1	0	1	127	5	12
Sopressata, Boar's Head	1 oz.	0	0	0	100	8	8

Food	Serving size	Carbohy-drates	Fiber	Net Carbs	Calories	Protein	Fat
Spam, Hormel	2 oz.	2	0	2	174	7	15
Turkey breast, roasted	1 oz.	0	0	0	24	4	0
Turkey breast, roasted, Boar's Head	2 oz.	0	0	0	60	13	1
Turkey breast, roasted, Cajun, Boar's Head	2 oz.	1	0	1	60	13	1
Turkey breast, roasted, pepper, Boar's Head	2 oz.	0	0	0	60	13	1
Turkey breast, roasted, Salsalito, Boar's Head	2 oz.	1	0	1	60	13	1
Turkey breast, smoked	2 oz.	1	0	1	52	11	0
Turkey breast, smoked, Boar's Head	2 oz.	1	0	1	60	13	1
Turkey roll	1 oz.	1	0	1	85	10	4
Vienna sausage	0.6 oz.	0	0	0	45	2	4

CONDIMENTS AND SAUCES

Flavorful additions that perk up ordinary foods, condiments such as mustard and ketchup are kitchen staples. Most are very low in carbs. Even the ones that contain more carbs are acceptable, as long as you stick to small amounts just to flavor your food. Tomato sauce, alfredo sauce, and other sauces also qualify as kitchen essentials. Here too, you can continue to enjoy these foods—just keep an eye on the carbs, and try the reduced-carb versions of favorite condiments and sauces.

Spices such as pepper, oregano, cinnamon, and so on contain small amounts of carbs. In general, the amounts used to season foods are so insignificant that they add no carbs to a portion.

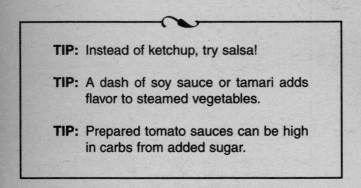

TIP: Instead of ketchup, try salsa!

TIP: A dash of soy sauce or tamari adds flavor to steamed vegetables.

TIP: Prepared tomato sauces can be high in carbs from added sugar.

Food	Serving size	Carbohy-drates	Fiber	Net Carbs	Calories	Protein	Fat
Alfredo sauce, Classico	½ cup	6	0	6	238	4	22
Alfredo sauce, Francesco Rinaldi	¼ cup	3	0	3	80	1	6
Alfredo, sundried tomato sauce, Classico	½ cup	8	4	4	228	4	20
Barbeque sauce, original, Bull's-Eye	2 T	15	0	15	63	0	0
Barbeque sauce, original, Kraft	2 T	9	0	9	39	0	0
Clam sauce, creamy, Progresso	½ cup	8	0	8	110	5	6
Clam sauce, red, Progresso	½ cup	8	0	8	60	4	1
Dijonnaise, Hellman's	1 t	1	0	1	5	0	0
Enchilada sauce, Old El Paso	¼ cup	3	0	3	20	0	1
Enchilada sauce, Ortega	2 T	2	0	2	15	0	1
Fish sauce	1 T	1	0	1	10	1	0
Hoisin sauce	1 T	7	0	7	35	0	0
Hollandaise sauce	1 oz.	9	0	9	157	3	13
Honey mustard dressing, Hellman's	1 t	1	0	1	10	0	0
Horseradish	1 t	0	0	0	0	0	0
Horseradish sauce	1 t	1	0	1	15	0	2
Ketchup, Heinz	1 T	4	0	4	16	0	0

Food	Serving size	Carbohy-drates	Fiber	Net Carbs	Calories	Protein	Fat
Marinara sauce, Francesco Rinaldi	½ cup	11	3	8	90	2	4
Marinara sauce, Prego	½ cup	11	4	7	100	2	5
Mustard, deli style	1 t	0	0	0	0	0	0
Mustard, honey	1 t	2	0	2	10	0	0
Mustard, yellow	1 t	0	0	0	3	0	0
Oyster sauce	1 T	2	0	2	9	0	0
pasta sauce, Italian sausage, garlic, Prego	½ cup	16	3	13	120	3	5
Pasta sauce, mushrooms, green peppers, Prego	½ cup	17	4	13	110	2	4
Pasta sauce, pesto, sundried tomato	¼ cup	8	1	7	89	3	5
Pasta sauce, tomato, pepper, Newman's Own	½ cup	9	0	9	40	0	2
Pasta sauce, traditional, Prego	½ cup	19	3	16	120	2	4
Pepper sauce, Tabasco	1 t	0	0	0	1	0	0
Picante sauce, Old El Paso	2 T	2	0	2	10	0	0
Picante sauce, Ortega	2 T	2	0	2	10	0	0
Plum sauce	1 T	8	0	8	35	0	0

Food	Serving size	Carbohydrates	Fiber	Net Carbs	Calories	Protein	Fat
Puttanesca sauce, Francesco Rinaldi	½ cup	8	0	8	70	2	4
Salsa	1 T	1	0	1	4	0	0
Salsa, Old El Paso	2 T	2	0	2	10	0	0
Salsa, thick, Old El Paso	2 T	3	0	3	10	0	0
Shoyu sauce	1 T	1	0	1	9	1	0
Soy sauce	1 T	1	0	1	11	2	0
Steak sauce, original, A-1	1 T	3	0	3	12	0	0
Steak sauce, Heinz	1 T	2	0	2	9	0	0
Steak sauce, Lawry's	1 T	3	0	3	12	0	0
Taco sauce, Old El Paso	1 T	1	0	1	5	0	0
Tamari sauce	1 T	1	0	1	11	2	0
Tartar sauce, Hellman's	2 T	3	0	3	80	0	7
Teriyaki sauce	1 T	3	0	3	15	0	0
Tomato basil sauce, Muir Glen	½ cup	12	0	12	65	2	1
Tomato basil sauce, Rinaldi	½ cup	11	0	11	80	4	3
Tomato sauce, Bertolli	½ cup	11	3	8	82	3	3
Tomato sauce, Progresso	½ cup	8	2	6	40	2	0

Food	Serving size	Carbohy-drates	Fiber	Net Carbs	Calories	Protein	Fat
Tomato sauce, Ragu Robusto	½ cup	10	2	8	87	3	4
Tomato sauce, original, Francesco Rinaldi	½ cup	11	3	8	90	2	4
Vodka sauce, Francesco Rinaldi	¼ cup	4	0	4	80	2	4

REDUCED-CARB PRODUCTS

Food	Serving size	Carbohy-drates	Fiber	Net Carbs	Calories	Protein	Fat
Alfredo sauce, Carb Options	¼ cup	2	0	2	110	1	10
Asian teriyaki marinade, Carb Options	1 T	1	0	1	5	0	0
Barbeque sauce, hickory, Carb Options	2 T	3	0	3	10	0	0
Barbecue sauce, original, Carb Options	2 T	3	0	3	10	0	0
Double cheddar sauce, Carb Options	¼ cup	2	0	2	90	2	8
Garden style sauce, Carb Options	½ cup	7	2	5	80	2	5
Hoisin sauce, Atkins	2 T	2	1	1	15	0	0
Hollandaise sauce, Atkins	2 T	0	0	0	100	0	11
Italian garlic marinade, Carb Options	1 T	0	0	0	0	0	0
Ketchup, Carb Options	1 T	0	0	0	5	0	0
Ketchup, Heinz One Carb	1 T	1	0	1	5	0	0

Food	Serving size	Carbohy-drates	Fiber	Net Carbs	Calories	Protein	Fat
Portobello mushroom sauce, Carb Fit	½ cup	7	2	5	60	2	3
Steak sauce, Atkins	1 T	1	0	1	5	0	0
Steak sauce, Carb Options	1 T	1	0	1	5	0	0
Sweet and sour sauce, Atkins	1 T	1	0	1	5	0	0
Tomato basil sauce, Carb Fit	½ cup	7	2	5	60	2	3
Vodka sauce, Carb Fit	½ cup	7	2	5	100	2	3

COOKIES

Few treats have as much comfort value as cookies—and few treats have as many carbs. Even worse, the carbs come almost entirely from highly refined ingredients such as white flour and sugar. Fortunately, most low-carb dieters find that when they start eating more whole grains and fresh fruits and vegetables, they quickly lose their taste for cookies. Save them for an occasional treat.

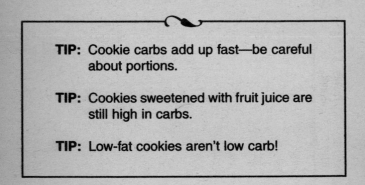

TIP: Cookie carbs add up fast—be careful about portions.

TIP: Cookies sweetened with fruit juice are still high in carbs.

TIP: Low-fat cookies aren't low carb!

Food	Serving size	Carbohy-drates	Fiber	Net Carbs	Calories	Protein	Fat
Animal crackers	2 oz.	42	1	41	254	4	8
Anisette toast	3 cookies	27	0	27	130	2	1
Apple 'n raisin, Archway	1 cookie	17	1	16	111	1	4
Arrowroot	1 cookie	4	0	4	22	0	0
Bordeaux, Pepperidge Farm	1 cookie	7	0	7	60	1	3
Brown-edge wafers, Nabisco	5 cookies	21	0	21	140	1	6
Brussels, Pepperidge Farm	1 cookie	7	0	7	43	1	2
Butter Chessmen	1 cookie	6	0	6	40	1	2
Butter	1 oz.	20	0	20	132	2	5
Cameo, Nabisco	3 cookies	40	0	40	250	1	9
Chips Ahoy, Nabisco	1 cookie	21	1	20	160	2	8
Chocolate chip, homemade	1 cookie	9	0	9	78	1	5
Chocolate chip, Chips Deluxe, Keebler	1 cookie	9	0	9	80	1	5
Chocolate chip, Soft Batch, Keebler	1 cookie	10	0	10	80	1	4
Chocolate Chunk Nantucket, Pepperidge Farm	1 cookie	16	0	16	135	2	7
Chocolate chunk pecan, Pepperidge Farm	1 cookie	8	0	8	58	1	3

Food	Serving size	Carbohy-drates	Fiber	Net Carbs	Calories	Protein	Fat
Chocolate wafers, Nabisco	5 cookies	21	1	20	123	2	4
Cinnamon apple, Archway	1 cookie	17	0	17	106	1	4
Coconut macaroon, Archway	1 cookie	12	0	12	106	1	6
Dutch cocoa, Archway	1 cookie	17	1	16	98	1	3
E.L. Fudge, Keebler	1 cookie	9	1	8	61	1	3
Fig Newtons, Nabisco	2 cookies	22	1	21	110	1	3
Frosty lemon, Archway	1 cookie	17	0	17	112	1	4
Fruit and honey bar, Archway	1 cookie	18	1	17	103	.1	3
Fudge sticks, Keebler	3 cookies	19	0	19	150	1	8
Gingersnaps	1 cookie	5	0	5	29	0	1
Gingersnaps, Keebler	5 cookies	24	0	24	150	2	6
Graham crackers, chocolate-coated	1 cookie	9	0	9	68	1	3
Graham crackers, chocolate-coated, Keebler	3 cookies	19	0	19	126	2	5
Graham crackers, cinnamon	5 cookies	26	0	26	140	2	3
Graham crackers, fudge, Keebler	3 cookies	19	0	19	140	1	7
Graham crackers, honey	2 cookies	11	0	11	59	1	1

Food	Serving size	Carbohy-drates	Fiber	Net Carbs	Calories	Protein	Fat
Grasshopper, Keebler	4 cookies	19	0	19	150	2	7
Hermits, Archway	1 cookie	17	1	16	95	1	3
Ladyfinger	1 cookie	7	0	7	40	1	1
Lorna Doone, Nabisco	4 cookies	19	0	19	140	2	7
Mallomars, Nabisco	2 cookies	17	0	17	120	1	5
Milano, Pepperidge Farm	1 cookie	7	0	7	60	1	3
Molasses	1 cookie	24	0	24	138	2	4
Molasses, Archway	1 cookie	18	0	18	103	1	3
Mystic Mint, Nabisco	1 cookie	11	0	11	90	1	4
Nilla Wafers, Nabisco	8 cookies	24	0	24	140	2	5
Nutter Butter, Nabisco	2 cookies	19	0	19	130	2	6
Oatmeal	1 cookie	12	1	11	81	1	3
Oatmeal, Archway	1 cookie	17	1	16	106	2	4
Oatmeal raisin	1 cookie	10	0	10	65	1	2
Oatmeal raisin, Archway	1 cookie	18	1	17	107	2	4
Oreo, Nabisco	3 cookies	24	2	23	167	2	7
Oreo Double Stuf, Nabisco	2 cookies	19	1	18	140	0	7

Food	Serving size	Carbohy-drates	Fiber	Net Carbs	Calories	Protein	Fat
Peanut butter	1 cookie	9	0	9	72	1	4
Peanut butter, Archway	1 cookie	12	1	11	101	2	5
Pecan shortbread	1 cookie	8	0	8	76	1	5
Pecan Shortbread Sandies, Keebler	1 cookie	9	0	9	80	1	5
Pinwheels, Nabisco	1 cookie	21	0	21	130	1	5
Raisin	1 cookie	10	0	10	60	1	2
Santa Fe, Pepperidge Farm	1 cookie	18	0	18	120	2	5
Sausalito, Pepperidge Farm	1 cookie	16	0	16	144	2	8
Shortbread	1 cookie	5	0	5	40	1	2
Social Tea Biscuits, Nabisco	1 cookie	3	0	3	18	0	1
Sugar	1 cookie	10	0	10	72	1	3
Sugar, Archway	1 cookie	17	0	17	98	1	3
Teddy Grahams, Nabisco	1 cookie	1	0	1	6	0	0
Vanilla wafers, Keebler	8 cookies	22	0	22	147	2	6
Vienna Fingers, Nabisco	2 cookies	21	0	21	140	2	6

Food	Serving size	Carbohy-drates	Fiber	Sugar Alcohol	Net Carbs	Calories	Protein	Fat
REDUCED-CARB PRODUCTS								
Almond, Health Valley Carb Fit	2 cookies	12	3	3	6	110	3	8
Chocolate caramel, Atkins	2 cookies	16	4	8	4	120	2	7
Chocolate chip, Atkins	6 cookies	22	8	8	6	170	5	11
Chocolate chip, Health Valley Carb Fit	2 cookies	12	3	2	7	110	3	8
Chocolate chip, sugar-free, Archway	1 cookie	16	0	0	16	108	1	5
Chocolate fudge, Atkins	2 cookies	16	5	7	4	120	2	7
Chocolate mint, Atkins	2 cookies	16	4	8	4	120	2	6
Chocolate raspberry, Atkins	2 cookies	18	8	5	5	90	2	4
Grahams, fudge-covered, CarbWell	2 cookies	18	1	11	6	139	1	7
Oatmeal, sugar-free, Archway	1 cookie	16	1	0	15	106	1	5
Oreo, CarbWell	2 cookies	16	3	7	6	100	2	5
Peanut butter, Health Valley Carb Fit	2 cookies	11	3	2	6	110	4	8
Rocky Road, sugar-free, Archway	1 cookie	16	1	0	15	101	1	5
Shortbread, sugar-free, Archway	1 cookie	16	0	0	16	107	1	5

CRACKERS

Crispy, crunchy crackers can still be an enjoyable part of your low-carb diet. Many cracker products are high in un-desirable refined carbs and trans fats, but today many others are made with whole grains and are fairly low in carbs. Choose the lower-carb brands—they make a good substitute for high-carb bread and rolls.

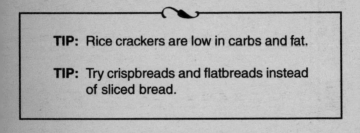

TIP: Rice crackers are low in carbs and fat.

TIP: Try crispbreads and flatbreads instead of sliced bread.

Food	Serving size	Carbohy-drates	Fiber	Net Carbs	Calories	Protein	Fat
Better Cheddars	22 crackers	18	0	18	150	0	7
Big Town	10 crackers	39	0	39	237	3	8
Brown rice, Eden	10 crackers	22	2	20	118	3	2
Brown rice snaps	8 crackers	11	1	10	50	1	0
Cheese, Snackwell's	15 crackers	11	0	11	60	2	1
Cheese Nips	32 crackers	21	0	21	130	3	4
Cheez-It	15 crackers	16	0	15	160	4	8
Chicken in a Biskit	12 crackers	17	0	17	160	0	9
Club	4 crackers	9	0	9	70	1	3
Finn Crisp	3 crackers	11	3	8	60	2	0
Flatbread, country onion, Atkins	3 crackers	8	4	4	140	10	8
Flatbread, Old World rye, Atkins	3 crackers	8	4	4	140	10	8
Flatbread, plain, Atkins	3 crackers	8	4	4	140	10	8
Flatbread, toasted sesame, Atkins	3 crackers	8	4	4	140	10	8
Crown Pilot	1 cracker	13	0	13	70	1	2
Garden Crisps	15 crackers	22	0	22	130	2	4
Harvest Crisps	13 crackers	23	0	23	130	3	4

Food	Serving size	Carbohy- drates	Fiber	Net Carbs	Calories	Protein	Fat
Hi Ho	5 crackers	10	0	10	70	1	4
Kavli Crispy Thin	3 crackers	13	2	11	60	1	0
Matzo, plain	½ matzo	12	0	12	56	1	0
Melba toast	2 crackers	8	1	7	39	1	0
Milk	1 cracker	8	0	8	50	1	2
Nori maki rice, Eden	10 crackers	16	1	15	70	2	0
Oat Thins	18 crackers	20	2	18	140	3	6
Oyster	23 crackers	11	0	11	60	1	2
Rice crackers	5 crackers	2	0	2	9	0	0
Ritz	5 crackers	10	0	10	80	1	4
Ritz Bitz sandwiches, cheese	14 crackers	17	0	17	160	3	10
Ritz Bitz sandwiches, peanut butter	13 crackers	17	0	17	150	4	8
Royal Lunch	15 crackers	8	0	8	50	1	2
Rye crispbread	1 cracker	8	2	6	37	1	0
Ryvita	2 crackers	14	3	11	60	2	0
Saltines	5 crackers	11	0	11	65	1	2
Sesame, Atkins	2 crackers	4	0	4	45	0	3

Food	Serving size	Carbohydrates	Fiber	Net Carbs	Calories	Protein	Fat
Sociables	7 crackers	9	0	9	80	1	4
Toasteds, wheat	10 crackers	18	1	17	130	2	6
Town House, original	10 crackers	18	1	17	160	2	9
Town House, wheat	10 crackers	18	1	17	160	2	9
Triscuit	6 crackers	18	3	15	128	3	6
Uneeda	2 crackers	11	0	11	65	1	2
Vegetable Thins	14 crackers	19	0	19	160	2	9
Wasa Crisp	2 crackers	10	5	5	62	2	0
Wasa Hearty Rye crispbread	2 crackers	18	4	14	90	2	0
Wasa Hearty Whole Grain crispbread	2 crackers	18	5	13	86	3	0
Wasa Sesame crispbread	2 crackers	17	2	15	112	3	3
Water biscuits, Carr's	5 crackers	13	1	12	70	2	2
Water biscuits, Pepperidge Farm	4 crackers	11	0	11	61	2	1
Waverly	5 crackers	10	0	10	70	1	4
Wheatables	16 crackers	20	0	20	140	2	6
Wheat Thins	16 crackers	20	1	19	136	2	6
Wheat, Snackwell's	15 crackers	11	0	11	70	2	2

Food	Serving size	Carbohy-drates	Fiber	Net Carbs	Calories	Protein	Fat
Wheatsworth	5 crackers	10	1	9	80	2	4
Whole wheat, Atkins	2 crackers	4	0	4	45	0	3
Whole wheat, Carr's	2 crackers	11	0	11	80	1	4
Zesta	2 crackers	4	0	4	26	1	1
Zwieback	1 cracker	6	0	6	35	1	1

EGGS AND EGG SUBSTITUTES

Eggs are the low-carb dieter's best friend. They're almost carb free, and also inexpensive, versatile, and very quick and easy to cook. Eggs are an excellent source of protein—in fact, eggs are the standard dietitians use when comparing the quality of different kinds of dietary protein. Eggs are also a good source of iron and vitamin A, among other important nutrients.

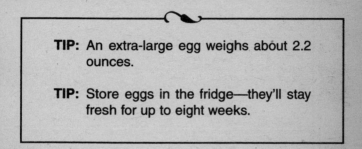

TIP: An extra-large egg weighs about 2.2 ounces.

TIP: Store eggs in the fridge—they'll stay fresh for up to eight weeks.

Food	Serving size	Carbohy-drates	Fiber	Net Carbs	Calories	Protein	Fat
Egg, hard/soft boiled	1 large egg	0.5	0	0.5	78	6	5
Egg, fried	1 large egg	0.5	0	0.5	92	6	7
Egg, poached	1 large egg	0.5	0	0.5	75	6	5
Egg, scrambled	1 large egg	0.5	0	0.5	93	6	7
Egg, white only	1 large egg	0	0	0	17	4	0
Egg, yolk only	1 large egg	0.5	0	0.5	61	3	5
Egg substitute, Morningstar Farms	2 oz.	0	0	0	26	5	0
Egg substitute, Egg Beaters	¼ cup	1	0	1	30	6	0

ENERGY, MEAL REPLACEMENT, AND SNACK BARS

For those times when a low-carb meal just isn't an option, choosing one of the many energy bars on the market can be a good alternative. While some bars are meant as snacks and are little different from candy, others are more substantial and are designed to be occasional meal replacements. Read the label carefully and select the bar that's best for you.

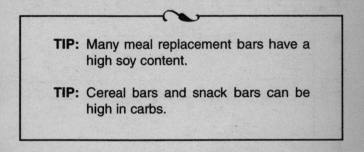

TIP: Many meal replacement bars have a high soy content.

TIP: Cereal bars and snack bars can be high in carbs.

Food	Serving size	Carbohy-drates	Fiber	Net Carbs	Calories	Protein	Fat
All-Bran, brown sugar cinnamon, Kellogg's	1 bar	27	5	22	130	2	3
All-Bran, honey oat, Kellogg's	1 bar	27	5	22	130	2	3
Balance Bar, chocolate	1 bar	22	0	22	200	14	6
Balance Bar, peanut butter	1 bar	22	1	21	200	14	6
Cereal, apple cinnamon, Nutri-Grain	1 bar	27	1	26	140	2	3
Cereal, blueberry, Nutri-Grain	1 bar	27	1	26	140	2	3
Cereal, Chex	1 bar	26	0	26	160	6	4
Cereal, Cocoa Puffs	1 bar	26	1	25	160	6	4
Cereal, Honey Nut Cheerios	1 bar	26	1	25	160	6	4
Cereal, mixed berry, Nutri-Grain	1 bar	27	1	26	140	2	3
Cereal, raspberry, Nutri-Grain	1 bar	27	1	26	140	2	3
Cereal, strawberry, Nutri-Grain	1 bar	27	1	26	140	2	3
Ensure, all flavors	1 bar	35	1	34	230	9	6
Granola, almond	1 bar	15	1	14	119	2	6
Granola, apple crisp, Quaker	1 bar	15	5	10	91	1	3
Granola, chocolate chip	1 bar	17	1	16	105	2	4
Granola, chocolate chip, chewy	1 bar	19	1	18	118	2	5

Food	Serving size	Carbohy-drates	Fiber	Net Carbs	Calories	Protein	Fat
Granola, chocolate chip, chewy, Quaker	1 bar	21	1	20	124	1	4
Granola, chocolate chip, Chewy Dipps	1 bar	21	1	20	146	2	6
Granola, chocolate chunk, Nutri-Grain	1 bar	17	0	17	100	2	4
Granola, cinnamon raisin, Nature's Choice	1 bar	14	0	14	80	2	2
Granola, cranberry, raisin, almond, Chewy Trail Mix	1 bar	24	1	23	153	3	5
Granola, crunchy, Nature's Choice	1 bar	15	1	14	90	2	3
Granola, honey oat and raisin, Nutri-Grain	1 bar	18	1	17	110	2	3
Granola, mixed nuts, Chewy Trail Mix	1 bar	23	1	22	158	3	6
Granola, nut and raisin, chewy	1 bar	18	2	16	127	2	6
Granola, peanut butter, Chewy Dipps	1 bar	18	1	17	147	3	7
Granola, peanut butter, chewy, Quaker	1 bar	20	1	19	124	3	4
Granola, plain	1 bar	18	2	16	132	3	6
Granola, plain, chewy	1 bar	19	1	18	124	2	5
Granola, raisin, chewy	1 bar	19	1	18	125	2	5
Granola, strawberry, Quaker	1 bar	26	1	25	135	1	3
Granola, very berry, Quaker	1 bar	26	1	25	135	1	3

Food	Serving size	Carbohydrates	Fiber	Net Carbs	Calories	Protein	Fat
Jenny Craig, chocolate peanut	1 bar	33	1	32	220	10	5
Jenny Craig, lemon meringue	1 bar	31	0	31	210	10	5
Jenny Craig, milk chocolate	1 bar	33	1	32	210	10	5
Jenny Craig, oatmeal raisin	1 bar	35	3	32	210	10	3
Jenny Craig, yogurt peanut	1 bar	33	1	32	220	10	5
Slim-Fast breakfast, cinnamon bun	1 bar	22	1	21	182	10	6
Slim-Fast breakfast, mixed berry	1 bar	22	1	21	182	10	6
Slim-Fast, caramel	1 bar	22	2	20	128	1	4
Slim-Fast, carrot cake	1 bar	25	1	24	214	15	6
Slim-Fast, oatmeal raisin	1 bar	35	2	33	217	8	5
SmartZone, chocolate	1 bar	21	3	18	210	14	8
SmartZone, lemon	1 bar	21	2	19	200	15	7
SmartZone, peanut butter chocolate	1 bar	20	3	17	210	15	8
SmartZone, strawberry	1 bar	22	2	20	200	14	7

Food	Serving size	Carbohy-drates	Fiber	Sugar Alcohol	Net Carbs	Calories	Protein	Fat
REDUCED-CARB PRODUCTS								
Atkins Advantage, almond brownie	1 bar	21	7	12	2	220	21	8
Atkins Advantage, chocolate	1 bar	21	9	10	2	230	19	11
Atkins Advantage, chocolate decadence	1 bar	25	11	12	2	220	17	11
Atkins Advantage, chocolate mocha crunch	1 bar	22	10	9	3	220	20	10
Atkins Advantage, chocolate peanut butter	1 bar	21	10	9	2	240	19	12
Atkins Advantage, cookies 'n creme	1 bar	22	11	9	2	220	18	11
Atkins Advantage, praline 'n creme	1 bar	18	7	8	3	250	21	13
Atkins Advantage, s'mores	1 bar	26	11	14	3	220	17	10
Carb Options, chocolate chip	1 bar	17	0	13	4	200	16	8
Carb Options, chocolate peanut	1 bar	17	0	13	4	200	16	8
Carb Options, cinnamon delight	1 bar	17	0	14	3	200	16	8
Carb Solutions, blueberry crumb pie	1 bar	24	2	16	4	200	13	9
Carb Solutions, cinnamon apple crisp	1 bar	14	0	8	6	150	13	6
Carb Solutions, creamy chocolate peanut butter	1 bar	14	1	10	3	250	23	12
Carb Solutions, fudge almond brownie	1 bar	15	1	11	3	240	23	11

Food	Serving size	Carbohy-drates	Fiber	Sugar Alcohol	Net Carbs	Calories	Protein	Fat
Power Bar Carb Select, chocolate caramel	1 bar	32	2	28	2	270	20	11
Power Bar Carb Select, chocolate peanut butter	1 bar	30	2	26	2	270	22	9
Power Bar Carb Select, double chocolate	1 bar	30	1	27	2	260	22	7
Power Bar Carb Select, peanut caramel	1 bar	32	1	29	2	270	20	11
Slim-Fast, banana nut	1 bar	18	1	0	17	123	6	3
Slim-Fast, caramel nut	1 bar	19	1	0	18	129	2	5
Slim-Fast, chocolate peanut	1 bar	18	1	0	17	123	6	3
Slim-Fast coconut almond	1 bar	15	2	0	13	129	6	5
Slim-Fast cookies n' cream	1 bar	18	1	0	17	123	6	3

FAST FOOD

Eating in fast food restaurants can be a real problem for someone trying to cut carbs. Those delicious french fries and creamy shakes are hard to resist, especially when there aren't many alternatives. But even when eating fast food is unavoidable, you can still make the best choices possible. Select the smallest portions, look for lower-carb options such as salads, and choose diet beverages.

TIP: Breakfast sandwiches tend to be very high in carbs.

TIP: Ask for the smallest serving of high-carb foods.

TIP: Some fast food restaurants offer bun-less burgers.

TIP: Choose roasted chicken instead of fried.

TIP: Sauces, condiments, and dressings can add carbs.

TIP: Ask for a side salad instead of fries.

TIP: Have a diet soda, not a shake.

TIP: Look for special low-carb menu items.

ARBY'S

Food	Serving size	Carbohy-drates	Fiber	Net Carbs	Calories	Protein	Fat
Arby-Q	1 sandwich	51	2	49	360	18	11
Beef 'n Cheddar	1 sandwich	44	2	42	440	22	21
Big Montana	1 sandwich	41	3	38	590	47	29
Chicken Bacon 'n Swiss	1 sandwich	49	2	47	550	31	27
Chicken Breast Fillet	1 sandwich	46	2	44	490	25	24
Chicken Club Wrap	1 sandwich	52	31	21	680	43	38
Chicken Cordon Bleu	1 sandwich	46	2	44	570	34	29
Chicken Fingers	4 pieces	42	3	39	640	31	38
French Dip 'n Swiss	1 sandwich	56	3	53	580	35	25
Giant Roast Beef	1 sandwich	41	2	39	450	32	19
Grilled Chicken Deluxe	1 sandwich	40	2	38	380	29	12
Hot Ham 'n Cheese	1 sandwich	35	1	34	300	23	9
Hot Ham 'n Swiss Melt	1 sandwich	35	1	34	270	18	8
Junior Roast Beef	1 sandwich	34	2	32	270	16	9
Market Fresh Chicken Salad	1 sandwich	92	6	86	860	26	44

Food	Serving size	Carbohydrates	Fiber	Net Carbs	Calories	Protein	Fat
Market Fresh Low Carbys Chicken Caesar Wrap	1 sandwich	46	30	16	520	33	27
Market Fresh Low Carbys Roast Turkey Ranch Bacon Wrap	1 sandwich	48	30	18	710	51	39
Market Fresh Low Carbys Southwest Chicken Wrap	1 sandwich	45	30	15	550	35	30
Market Fresh Low Carbys Ultimate BLT Wrap	1 sandwich	48	31	17	650	25	47
Market Fresh Roast Beef and Swiss	1 sandwich	74	6	68	789	37	39
Market Fresh Roast Ham and Swiss	1 sandwich	74	5	69	700	36	31
Market Fresh Roast Turkey, Ranch, Bacon	1 sandwich	75	5	70	830	49	38
Market Fresh Roast Turkey and Swiss	1 sandwich	74	5	69	720	45	27
Market Fresh Ultimate BLT	1 sandwich	75	6	69	780	23	46
Philly Beef Supreme	1 sandwich	59	3	56	450	36	37
Regular Roast Beef	1 sandwich	34	2	32	320	21	13
Roast Chicken Club	1 sandwich	39	2	37	470	27	25
Super Roast Beef	1 sandwich	48	3	45	440	22	19

Food	Serving size	Carbohy-drates	Fiber	Net Carbs	Calories	Protein	Fat
BURGER KING							
Angus Bacon & Cheese	1 sandwich	64	3	61	710	41	33
Angus Steak Burger	1 sandwich	62	3	59	570	33	22
Bacon cheeseburger	1 sandwich	31	1	30	390	22	20
Bacon double cheeseburger	1 sandwich	32	2	30	570	35	34
BK Fish Filet	1 sandwich	44	2	42	520	18	30
BK Veggie Burger	1 sandwich	46	4	42	380	14	16
Cheeseburger	1 sandwich	31	1	30	350	19	17
Chicken Caesar salad, no dressing	1 salad	9	1	8	190	25	7
Chicken garden salad, no dressing	1 salad	12	2	10	210	26	7
Chicken, original	1 sandwich	52	3	49	560	25	28
Chicken Tenders	6 pieces	15	0	15	250	18	14
Chicken Whopper	1 sandwich	48	4	44	570	38	25
Chili	1 cup	17	5	12	190	13	8
Croissan'wich, bacon, egg, cheese	1 sandwich	25	0	25	360	15	22
Croissan'wich, egg, cheese	1 sandwich	24	0	24	320	12	19
Croissan'wich, ham, egg, cheese	1 sandwich	25	0	25	360	18	20

Food	Serving size	Carbohy-drates	Fiber	Net Carbs	Calories	Protein	Fat
Croissan'wich, sausage, cheese	1 sandwich	23	0	23	420	14	31
Croissan'wich, sausage, egg, cheese	1 sandwich	24	1	23	520	19	39
Dipping sauce, barbecue	1 oz.	9	0	9	35	0	0
Dipping sauce, honey-flavored	1 oz.	23	0	23	90	0	0
Dipping sauce, honey mustard	1 oz.	9	0	9	90	0	0
Dipping sauce, ranch	1 oz.	1	0	1	140	1	15
Dipping sauce, sweet and sour	1 oz.	10	0	10	40	0	0
Dipping sauce, zesty onion ring	1 oz.	3	0	3	150	0	15
Double cheeseburger	1 sandwich	32	2	30	530	32	31
Double hamburger	1 sandwich	30	1	29	440	28	23
Double Whopper	1 sandwich	52	4	48	970	52	61
Double Whopper, cheese	1 sandwich	53	4	49	1060	56	69
Dressing, creamy garlic Caesar	2 oz.	7	0	7	130	2	11
Dressing, fat-free honey mustard	2 oz.	18	0	18	70	0	0
Dressing, garden ranch	2 oz.	7	0	7	120	0	10
Dressing, sweet onion vinaigrette	2 oz.	8	0	8	100	0	8
Dressing, tomato balsamic vinaigrette	2 oz.	9	0	9	110	0	9

	Serving size	Carbohy-drates	Fiber	Net Carbs	Calories	Protein	Fat
Apple pie	1 pie	52	1	51	340	2	14
fries	small	29	2	27	230	3	11
ench fries	medium	46	4	42	360	4	18
French fries	large	63	5	58	500	6	25
French fries	king	76	6	70	600	7	30
Garden salad, side, no dressing	1 salad	4	1	3	20	1	0
Hamburger	1 sandwich	30	1	29	310	17	13
Hershey's Sundae Pie	1 pie	31	1	30	300	3	18
Milk shake, chocolate	medium	97	2	95	600	2	18
Milk shake, strawberry	medium	96	0	96	590	9	17
Milk shake, vanilla	medium	76	0	76	540	11	20
Onion rings	small	22	2	20	180	2	9
Onion rings	medium	40	3	37	320	4	18
Onion rings	large	60	5	55	480	7	23
Onion rings	king	70	5	65	550	8	27
Shrimp Caesar salad, no dressing	1 salad	9	2	7	180	20	10
Shrimp garden salad, no dressing	1 salad	13	3	10	200	21	10

Food	Serving size	Carbohy-drates	Fiber	Net Carbs	Calories	Protein	Fat
TenderCrisp chicken	1 sandwich	70	6	74	780	27	45
TenderCrisp chicken, spicy	1 sandwich	71	6	65	720	27	38
Whopper	1 sandwich	52	4	48	700	31	42
Whopper, cheese	1 sandwich	53	4	49	800	35	49
Whopper Jr.	1 sandwich	31	2	29	390	31	22
Whopper Jr., cheese	1 sandwich	32	2	30	430	19	26
BURGER KING LOW-CARB CHOICES							
Angus Bacon & Cheese, low-carb	1 sandwich	7	0	7	420	33	29
Angus Steak Burger, low-carb	1 sandwich	5	0	5	280	25	18
Chicken Whopper, low-carb	1 sandwich	3	1	2	160	30	4
Double Whopper, low-carb	1 sandwich	3	0	3	540	43	40
Double Whopper, cheese, low-carb	1 sandwich	5	0	5	630	48	47
Whopper, low-carb	1 sandwich	3	0	3	280	22	20
Whopper, cheese, low-carb	1 sandwich	5	0	5	370	27	28
Whopper Jr., low-carb	1 sandwich	1	0	1	140	11	10
Whopper Jr., cheese, low-carb	1 sandwich	2	0	2	190	14	14

DAIRY QUEEN

Food	Serving size	Carbohy-drates	Fiber	Net Carbs	Calories	Protein	Fat
Blizzard, banana split	16 fl. oz.	97	1	96	580	12	17
Blizzard, chocolate chip cookie dough	16 fl. oz.	150	0	150	1030	17	40
Blizzard, Oreo	16 fl. oz.	103	1	102	700	13	26
Blizzard, Reese's Peanut Butter Cup	16 fl. oz.	114	0	114	790	18	28
Blizzard, Strawberry CheeseQuake	16 fl. oz.	105	0	105	730	13	29
Buster Bar	1 bar	45	2	43	500	11	28
Chocolate Dilly Bar	1 bar	25	0	25	220	3	13
Cone, chocolate	medium	53	0	53	340	8	7
Cone, vanilla	medium	53	0	53	330	8	9
Dipped cone	medium	59	1	58	490	8	24
DQ Fudge Bar	1 bar	13	0	13	50	0	0
DQ Sandwich	1 sandwich	31	1	30	200	4	6
DQ Vanilla Orange Bar	1 bar	17	0	17	60	2	0
Lemon DQ Freez'r	½ cup	20	0	20	80	0	0
Malt, chocolate	medium	153	2	151	870	20	22
Misty Slush	medium	74	0	74	290	0	0

Food	Serving size	Carbohy-drates	Fiber	Net Carbs	Calories	Protein	Fat
Moolatté, cappuccino	12 fl. oz.	68	0	68	490	7	18
Moolatté, French vanilla	12 fl. oz.	87	0	87	570	7	18
Moolatté, mocha	12 fl. oz.	80	1	79	590	8	23
Royal Treat, banana split	1 serving	96	3	93	510	8	12
Royal Treat, Brownie Earthquake	1 serving	112	0	112	740	10	27
Royal Treat, Peanut Buster parfait	1 serving	99	2	97	730	16	31
Royal Treat, strawberry shortcake	1 serving	70	1	69	430	7	14
Royal Treat, Triple Chocolate Utopia	1 serving	96	5	91	770	12	39
Shake, chocolate	medium	129	2	127	760	17	20
StarKiss	1 serving	21	0	21	80	0	0
Sundae, chocolate	medium	71	0	71	400	8	10
Sundae, strawberry	medium	58	0	58	340	7	9

DOMINO'S PIZZA

Food	Serving size	Carbohy-drates	Fiber	Net Carbs	Calories	Protein	Fat
America's Favorite Feast pizza, deep dish	1 large slice	42	3	39	433	17	8
America's Favorite Feast pizza, hand-tossed	1 large slice	39	2	37	353	14	16
America's Favorite Feast pizza, thin crust	1 large slice	20	2	18	285	11	7

Food	Serving size	Carbohy-drates	Fiber	Net Carbs	Calories	Protein	Fat
Bacon Cheeseburger Feast pizza, deep dish	1 large slice	41	2	39	459	20	26
Bacon Cheeseburger Feast pizza, hand-tossed	1 large slice	38	2	36	379	17	18
Bacon Cheeseburger Feast pizza, thin crust	1 large slice	19	1	18	311	14	21
Barbecue Feast pizza, deep dish	1 large slice	46	2	44	424	17	21
Barbecue Feast pizza, hand-tossed	1 large slice	43	2	41	344	14	14
Barbecue Feast pizza, thin crust	1 large slice	24	1	23	276	11	16
Beef pizza, deep dish	1 large slice	41	2	39	392	15	20
Beef pizza, hand-tossed	1 large slice	38	2	36	312	13	13
Beef pizza, thin crust	1 large slice	19	1	18	243	10	15
Cheese pizza, deep dish	1 large slice	41	2	39	336	13	15
Cheese pizza, hand-tossed	1 large slice	38	2	36	256	10	8
Cheese pizza, thin crust	1 large slice	19	1	18	188	7	10
Deluxe Feast pizza, deep dish	1 large slice	42	3	39	396	15	20
Deluxe Feast pizza, hand-tossed	1 large slice	39	3	37	316	13	13
Deluxe Feast pizza, thin crust	1 large slice	20	2	18	248	10	15
Extravaganzza Feast pizza, deep dish	1 large slice	43	3	40	468	20	10
Extravaganzza Feast pizza, hand-tossed	1 large slice	40	3	37	388	17	19

Food	Serving size	Carbohy-drates	Fiber	Net Carbs	Calories	Protein	Fat
Extravaganzza Feast pizza, thin crust	1 large slice	21	2	19	320	14	21
Green pepper, onion, mushroom pizza, deep dish	1 large slice	42	3	39	343	13	15
Green pepper, onion, mushroom pizza, hand-tossed	1 large slice	39	2	37	263	11	8
Green pepper, onion, mushroom pizza, thin crust	1 large slice	21	2	19	201	8	10
Ham pizza, deep dish	1 large slice	41	2	39	352	15	16
Ham pizza, hand-tossed	1 large slice	38	2	36	272	12	9
Ham pizza, thin crust	1 large slice	19	1	18	204	9	11
Ham, pineapple pizza, deep dish	1 large slice	42	2	40	355	14	16
Ham, pineapple pizza, hand-tossed	1 large slice	40	2	38	275	12	9
Ham, pineapple pizza, thin crust	1 large slice	21	1	20	207	9	11
Hawaiian Feast pizza, deep dish	1 large slice	43	3	40	389	17	18
Hawaiian Feast pizza, hand-tossed	1 large slice	41	2	39	309	14	11
Hawaiian Feast pizza, thin crust	1 large slice	21	2	19	240	11	13
Meatzza Feast pizza, deep dish	1 large slice	42	3	39	458	19	25

Food	Serving size	Carbohydrates	Fiber	Net Carbs	Calories	Protein	Fat
Meatzza Feast pizza, hand-tossed	1 large slice	35	2	33	378	17	18
Meatzza Feast pizza, thin crust	1 large slice	20	2	18	310	14	20
Pepperoni pizza, deep dish	1 large slice	41	2	39	385	15	20
Pepperoni pizza, hand-tossed	1 large slice	38	2	36	305	12	12
Pepperoni pizza, thin crust	1 large slice	19	1	18	237	10	15
Pepperoni Feast pizza, deep dish	1 large slice	42	3	39	443	18	24
Pepperoni Feast pizza, hand-tossed	1 large slice	39	2	37	363	16	17
Pepperoni Feast pizza, thin crust	1 large slice	28	1	27	295	18	19
Pepperoni, sausage pizza, deep dish	1 large slice	41	3	38	430	17	23
Pepperoni, sausage pizza, hand-tossed	1 large slice	39	2	37	350	14	16.
Pepperoni, sausage pizza, thin crust	1 large slice	19	2	17	282	11	7
Sausage pizza, deep dish	1 large slice	42	3	39	400	15	21
Sausage pizza, hand-tossed	1 large slice	39	2	37	320	13	14
Sausage pizza, thin crust	1 large slice	20	2	18	252	10	16
Vegi Feast pizza, deep dish	1 large slice	43	3	40	380	15	18
Vegi Feast pizza, hand-tossed	1 large slice	40	3	37	300	13	11
Vegi Feast pizza, thin crust	1 large slice	21	2	19	231	10	14

KFC

Food	Serving size	Carbohy-drates	Fiber	Net Carbs	Calories	Protein	Fat
Apple pie	1 serving	44	2	42	290	2	11
BBQ beans	1 serving	46	7	39	230	8	1
Biscuit	1 biscuit	23	0	23	190	2	10
BLT salad, no dressing	1 salad	8	4	4	210	28	7
Caesar salad, no dressing	1 salad	6	3	3	220	29	9
Chicken, extra-crispy, breast	1 serving	19	0	19	460	34	28
Chicken, extra-crispy, drumstick	1 serving	5	0	5	160	12	10
Chicken, extra-crispy, thigh	1 serving	12	0	12	370	21	26
Chicken, extra-crispy, wing	1 serving	10	0	10	190	10	12
Chicken, original, breast	1 serving	11	0	11	380	40	19
Chicken, original, breast, no breading	1 serving	0	0	0	140	29	3
Chicken, original, drumstick	1 serving	4	0	4	140	14	8
Chicken, original, thigh	1 serving	12	0	12	360	22	25
Chicken, original, wing	1 serving	5	0	5	150	11	9
Chicken pot pie	1 serving	70	5	65	770	33	40
Cole slaw	1 serving	22	3	19	190	1	11

Food	Serving size	Carbohy-drates	Fiber	Net Carbs	Calories	Protein	Fat
Corn on the cob	3" piece	13	3	10	70	2	2
Corn on the cob	5.5" piece	26	7	19	150	5	3
Crispy Strips	3 pieces	17	0	17	400	29	24
Double chocolate chip cake	1 serving	31	2	29	400	4	29
Green beans	1 serving	7	2	5	50	10	2
HBBQ sandwich	1 sandwich	41	4	37	300	21	6
HBBQ wings, sauce	6 pieces	36	1	35	540	25	33
Hot wings	6 pieces	23	1	22	450	24	29
Lemon meringue pie	1 serving	40	1	39	240	1	9
Lil' Bucket chocolate cream	1 serving	37	2	35	270	2	13
Lil' Bucket fudge brownie	1 serving	44	1	43	270	4	29
Lil' Bucket lemon crème	1 serving	65	2	63	400	4	14
Lil' Bucket strawberry short cake	1 serving	34	0	34	200	2	6
Mac and cheese	1 serving	45	4	41	400	15	18
Mashed potatoes	1 serving	16	1	15	110	2	4
Mashed potatoes, gravy	1 serving	18	1	17	120	2	5
Pecan pie	1 serving	68	2	66	480	5	21

Food	Serving size	Carbohy-drates	Fiber	Net Carbs	Calories	Protein	Fat
Popcorn chicken	1 serving	25	0	25	450	19	30
Potato salad	1 serving	22	1	21	180	2	9
Potato wedges	1 serving	30	3	27	240	4	12
Seasoned rice	1 serving	32	2	30	150	4	1
Sweet potato pie	1 serving	44	1	43	340	5	16
Tender Roast plated meal	1 serving	41	4	37	360	33	7
Tender Roast sandwich	1 sandwich	24	1	23	390	31	19
Tender Roast Twister	1 sandwich	50	4	46	510	29	22
Twister	1 sandwich	55	3	52	670	27	38

McDONALD'S

Food	Serving size	Carbohy-drates	Fiber	Net Carbs	Calories	Protein	Fat
Bacon, egg, cheese biscuit	1 sandwich	36	1	35	440	19	24
Bacon, egg, cheese McGriddles	1 serving	46	1	45	450	20	21
Bacon ranch salad	1 salad	8	3	5	130	9	7
Bacon ranch salad, crispy chicken	1 salad	23	3	20	340	27	16
Bacon ranch salad, grilled chicken	1 salad	11	3	8	240	31	9
Baked apple pie	1 serving	34	2	32	250	2	11

Food	Serving size	Carbohy-drates	Fiber	Net Carbs	Calories	Protein	Fat
Barbeque sauce	1 package	11	0	11	45	0	0
Big Breakfast	1 serving	53	3	50	730	27	46
Big Mac	1 sandwich	46	3	43	560	25	30
Big N' Tasty	1 sandwich	41	3	38	520	24	29
Big N' Tasty with cheese	1 sandwich	43	3	40	570	27	33
Biscuit	1 biscuit	31	1	30	240	4	11
Caesar salad	1 salad	7	3	4	90	6	4
Caesar salad, crispy chicken	1 salad	22	3	19	300	24	14
Caesar salad, grilled chicken	1 salad	10	3	7	200	28	6
California Cobb salad	1 salad	7	3	4	150	11	9
California Cobb salad, crispy chicken	1 salad	22	3	19	360	29	18
California Cobb salad, grilled chicken	1 salad	10	3	7	260	32	11
Cheeseburger	1 sandwich	35	1	34	310	15	12
Chicken McGrill	1 sandwich	38	3	35	400	27	16
Chicken McNuggets	4 pieces	10	0	10	170	10	10
Chicken McNuggets	6 pieces	15	0	15	250	15	15
Chicken McNuggets	10 pieces	26	0	26	420	25	24

Food	Serving size	Carbohy-drates	Fiber	Net Carbs	Calories	Protein	Fat
Chicken Selects	3 pieces	28	0	28	380	23	20
Chicken Selects	5 pieces	46	0	46	630	39	33
Chicken Selects	10 pieces	92	0	92	1270	77	66
Chocolate Triple Thick shake	12 fl. oz.	76	0	76	440	10	10
Chocolate Triple Thick shake	16 fl. oz.	102	0	102	580	13	14
Chocolate Triple Thick shake	21 fl. oz.	134	0	134	770	18	18
Chocolate Triple Thick shake	32 fl. oz.	203	0	203	1160	27	27
Cinnamon roll	1 roll	57	2	55	420	8	18
Creamy ranch sauce	1 package	3	0	3	200	0	21
Crispy Chicken	1 sandwich	50	3	47	500	24	23
Deluxe breakfast	1 serving	136	4	132	1220	33	60
Double cheeseburger	1 sandwich	37	1	36	210	25	23
Double Quarter-Pounder with cheese	1 sandwich	46	3	43	730	47	40
Egg McMuffin	1 sandwich	30	2	28	290	17	11
Fiesta salad, sour cream, salsa	1 salad	28	5	23	450	24	27
Filet-O-Fish	1 sandwich	42	1	41	400	14	18
French fries, large	6 oz.	70	7	63	520	6	25

Food	Serving size	Carbohy-drates	Fiber	Net Carbs	Calories	Protein	Fat
French fries, medium	4 oz.	47	5	42	350	4	16
French fries, small	2.6 oz.	30	3	27	230	2	11
Fruit 'n yogurt parfait.	1 serving	31	0	31	160	4	2
Hamburger	1 sandwich	33	1	32	260	13	9
Ham, egg, cheese bagel	1 sandwich	62	2	60	550	28	21
Hash browns	1 serving	15	2	13	140	1	8
Hotcakes	1 serving	102	2	100	600	9	17
Hotcakes and sausage	1 serving	104	2	102	770	15	33
Hot caramel sundae	1 serving	62	0	62	340	7	7
Hot fudge sundae	1 serving	55	0	55	330	8	9
Hot mustard sauce	1 package	9	1	8	50	1	2
Hot 'n Spicy McChicken	1 sandwich	42	1	41	440	14	24
M&Ms McFlurry	12 fl. oz.	96	0	96	620	14	20
McChicken	1 sandwich	41	1	40	420	15	22
McDonaldland chocolate chip cookies	1 package	39	1	38	270	3	11
McDonaldland cookies	1 package	42	0	42	250	4	8
Oreo McFlurry	12 fl. oz.	88	0	88	560	14	16

Food	Serving size	Carbohy-drates	Fiber	Net Carbs	Calories	Protein	Fat
Quarter-Pounder	1 sandwich	40	3	37	420	24	18
Quarter-Pounder with cheese	1 sandwich	43	3	40	510	29	25
Sausage biscuit	1 sandwich	34	1	33	410	10	26
Sausage biscuit, egg	1 sandwich	36	1	35	500	18	32
Sausage burrito	1 sandwich	26	1	25	300	13	16
Sausage, egg, cheese McGriddles	1 serving	48	1	47	560	21	32
Sausage McGriddles	1 serving	44	1	43	420	11	22
Sausage McMuffin	1 sandwich	31	2	29	370	14	21
Sausage McMuffin, egg	1 sandwich	31	2	29	450	20	26
Sausage patty	1 serving	2	0	2	170	7	15
Side salad	1 salad	3	1	2	15	1	0
Spanish omelet bagel	1 sandwich	64	3	1	710	29	38
Spicy Buffalo sauce	1 package	1	0	1	60	0	6
Steak, egg, cheese bagel	1 sandwich	61	2	59	640	33	29
Strawberry sundae	1 serving	51	0	51	280	6	6
Strawberry Triple Thick shake	12 fl. oz.	73	0	73	420	10	10
Strawberry Triple Thick shake	16 fl. oz.	97	0	97	560	13	13

Food	Serving size	Carbohy-drates	Fiber	Net Carbs	Calories	Protein	Fat
Strawberry Triple Thick shake	21 fl. oz.	128	0	128	740	17	17
Strawberry Triple Thick shake	32 fl. oz.	194	0	194	1110	25	26
Sweet 'n sour sauce	1 package	11	0	11	50	0	0
Tangy honey mustard sauce	1 package	13	1	12	70	1	3
Vanilla Triple Thick shake	12 fl. oz.	72	0	72	420	9	10
Vanilla Triple Thick shake	16 fl. oz.	96	0	96	550	13	13
Vanilla Triple Thick shake	21 fl. oz.	128	0	128	740	17	18
Vanilla Triple Thick shake	32 fl. oz.	193	0	193	1110	25	26

PIZZA HUT

Food	Serving size	Carbohy-drates	Fiber	Net Carbs	Calories	Protein	Fat
Apple dessert pizza	1 slice	53	1	52	260	4	4
Breadstick	1 piece	20	0	20	150	4	6
Cheese breadstick	1 piece	21	0	21	200	7	10
Cherry dessert pizza	1 slice	47	1	46	240	4	4
Cinnamon sticks	2 pieces	27	0	27	170	4	5
Fit 'n Delicious pizza, chicken, mushrooms	1 slice	22	2	20	170	10	5

Food	Serving size	Carbohydrates	Fiber	Net Carbs	Calories	Protein	Fat
Fit 'n Delicious pizza, chicken, onion, pepper	1 slice	23	2	21	170	10	5
Fit 'n Delicious pizza, ham, onion, mushroom	1 slice	22	2	20	160	8	5
Fit 'n Delicious pizza, ham, pineapple	1 slice	24	2	22	160	8	4
Fit 'n Delicious pizza, pepper, onion, tomato	1 slice	24	2	22	150	6	4
Fit 'n Delicious pizza, tomato, mushroom	1 slice	22	2	20	150	6	4
Pan Pizza, cheese	1 slice	29	1	28	280	11	13
Pan Pizza, Chicken Supreme	1 slice	30	2	28	280	13	12
Pan Pizza, Meat Lover's	1 slice	29	2	27	340	15	19
Pan Pizza, pepperoni	1 slice	29	2	27	290	11	15
Pan Pizza, Pepperoni Lover's	1 slice	29	2	27	340	15	19
Pan Pizza, quartered ham	1 slice	29	1	28	260	11	11
Pan Pizza, Sausage Lover's	1 slice	29	2	27	330	13	17
Pan Pizza, Super Supreme	1 slice	30	2	28	340	14	18
Pan Pizza, Supreme	1 slice	30	2	28	320	13	16
Pan Pizza, Veggie Lover's	1 slice	30	2	28	260	10	12

Food	Serving size	Carbohy-drates	Fiber	Net Carbs	Calories	Protein	Fat
P'zone, classic	½ P'zone	71	3	68	610	33	21
P'zone, Meat Lover's	½ P'zone	70	3	67	680	38	28
P'zone, pepperoni	½ P'zone	69	3	66	610	34	22
Stuffed Crust Pizza, cheese	1 slice	43	2	41	360	18	13
Stuffed Crust Pizza, Chicken Supreme	1 slice	44	3	41	380	20	13
Stuffed Crust Pizza, Meat Lover's	1 slice	443	3	40	450	21	21
Stuffed Crust Pizza, pepperoni	1 slice	42	3	39	370	18	15
Stuffed Crust Pizza, Pepperoni Lover's	1 slice	43	3	40	420	21	19
Stuffed Crust Pizza, quartered ham	1 slice	42	2	40	340	18	11
Stuffed Crust Pizza, Sausage Lover's	1 slice	43	3	40	430	19	19
Stuffed Crust Pizza, Super Supreme	1 slice	45	3	42	440	21	20
Stuffed Crust Pizza, Supreme	1 slice	44	3	41	400	20	16
Stuffed Crust Pizza, Veggie Lover's	1 slice	45	3	42	360	16	14
Thin 'n Crispy Pizza, cheese	1 slice	21	1	20	200	10	8
Thin 'n Crispy Pizza, Chicken Supreme	1 slice	22	1	21	200	12	7
Thin 'n Crispy Pizza, Meat Lover's	1 slice	21	2	19	270	13	14
Thin 'n Crispy Pizza, pepperoni	1 slice	21	1	20	210	10	10

Food	Serving size	Carbohy-drates	Fiber	Net Carbs	Calories	Protein	Fat
Thin 'n Crispy Pizza, Pepperoni Lover's	1 slice	21	2	19	260	13	14
Thin 'n Crispy Pizza, quartered ham	1 slice	21	1	20	180	9	6
Thin 'n Crispy Pizza, Sausage Lover's	1 slice	21	2	19	240	11	13
Thin 'n Crispy Pizza, Super Supreme	1 slice	23	2	21	240	13	13
Thin 'n Crispy Pizza, Supreme	1 slice	22	2	20	240	11	11
Thin 'n Crispy Pizza, Veggie Lover's	1 slice	23	2	21	180	8	7
Wings blue cheese sauce	1.5 oz.	2	0	2	230	2	24
Wings, hot	2 pieces	1	0	1	110	11	6
Wings, mild	2 pieces	0	0	0	110	11	7
Wings ranch sauce	1.5 oz.	4	0	4	210	0	22
SUBWAY							
Bacon, egg	1 deli sandwich	34	3	31	320	15	15
Bacon, egg	1 6" sandwich	42	3	39	450	28	19
Cheese, egg	1 deli sandwich	34	3	31	320	14	15
Cheese, egg	1 6" sandwich	42	3	39	440	27	19
Cheese steak	1 6" sandwich	47	5	42	360	24	10

Food	Serving size	Carbohy-drates	Fiber	Net Carbs	Calories	Protein	Fat
Chicken and bacon ranch	1 6" sandwich	48	5	43	640	43	34
Chicken and bacon ranch	1 wrap	18	9	9	440	41	27
Chipotle southwest cheese steak	1 6" sandwich	48	6	42	450	24	20
Classic tuna	1 6" sandwich	45	4	41	530	22	31
Classic tuna	1 deli sandwich	35	3	32	350	14	18
Cold cut combo	1 6" sandwich	47	4	43	410	47	17
Grilled chicken, spinach salad	1 salad	11	4	7	140	20	3
Ham	1 deli sandwich	36	3	33	210	11	4
Ham, egg	1 deli sandwich	34	3	31	310	16	13
Ham, egg	1 6" sandwich	42	3	39	430	29	17
Honey mustard ham	1 6" sandwich	53	4	49	320	18	5
Italian BMT	1 6" sandwich	47	4	43	450	23	21
Meatball marinara	1 6" sandwich	63	7	56	560	24	24
Oven roasted chicken breast	1 6" sandwich	47	4	43	330	24	5
Roast beef	1 6" sandwich	45	4	41	290	19	5
Roast beef	1 deli sandwich	35	3	32	220	13	5
Steak, egg	1 deli sandwich	35	3	32	330	19	14

Food	Serving size	Carbohydrates	Fiber	Net Carbs	Calories	Protein	Fat
Steak, egg	1 6" sandwich	43	4	39	460	33	18
Subway Club	1 6" sandwich	47	4	43	320	24	6
Subway Club salad	1 salad	15	4	11	160	18	4
Subway Seafood Sensation	1 6" sandwich	51	5	46	450	16	22
Sweet onion chicken teriyaki	1 6" sandwich	59	4	55	370	26	5
Tuna, cheese	1 wrap	16	9	7	440	27	32
Tuna, cheese salad	1 salad	12	4	8	360	16	29
Turkey breast	1 6" sandwich	46	4	42	280	18	5
Turkey breast	1 deli sandwich	36	3	33	210	13	4
Turkey breast	1 wrap	18	9	9	190	24	6
Turkey breast, bacon melt	1 wrap	20	9	11	440	34	28
Turkey breast, ham	1 6" sandwich	47	4	43	290	20	5
Turkey breast, ham, bacon melt	1 6" sandwich	48	4	44	380	25	12
Vegetable, egg	1 deli sandwich	36	3	33	290	12	12
Vegetable, egg	1 6" sandwich	44	4	40	410	25	16
Veggie Delite	1 6" sandwich	44	4	40	230	9	3
Veggie Delite salad	1 salad	12	4	8	60	3	1

	Serving size	Carbohy-drates	Fiber	Net Carbs	Calories	Protein	Fat
Western, egg	1 deli sandwich	36	3	33	300	14	12
Western, egg	1 6" sandwich	44	4	40	430	27	17
TACO BELL							
Bean burrito	1 burrito	55	8	47	370	14	10
Bean Burrito Especial	1 burrito	82	12	70	600	21	21
Bean burrito, fresco	1 burrito	56	9	47	350	13	8
Beef combo burrito	1 burrito	52	5	47	470	22	19
Beef, potato burrito	1 burrito	65	4	61	530	15	24
Burrito Supreme, beef	1 burrito	52	5	47	440	17	18
Burrito Supreme, chicken	1 burrito	50	5	45	410	21	14
Burrito Supreme, chicken, fresco	1 burrito	50	6	44	350	19	8
Burrito Supreme, steak	1 burrito	50	6	44	420	19	16
Burrito Supreme, steak, fresco	1 burrito	50	6	44	350	17	9
Caramel apple empanada	1 empanada	37	1	36	290	3	15
Chalupa Baja, beef	1 chalupa	32	2	30	430	13	27
Chalupa Baja, chicken	1 chalupa	30	2	28	400	17	24

Food	Serving size	Carbohy-drates	Fiber	Net Carbs	Calories	Protein	Fat
Chalupa nacho cheese, beef	1 chalupa	33	1	32	380	12	22
Chalupa nacho cheese, chicken	1 chalupa	31	1	30	350	16	18
Chalupa nacho cheese, steak	1 chalupa	31	2	29	350	14	19
Chalupa Baja, steak	1 chalupa	30	2	28	400	15	25
Chalupa Supreme, beef	1 chalupa	31	1	30	390	14	24
Chalupa Supreme, chicken	1 chalupa	30	1	29	370	17	20
Chalupa Supreme, steak	1 chalupa	29	2	27	370	15	22
Cheese quesadilla	1 quesadilla	39	3	36	490	19	28
Cheesy fiesta potatoes	1 serving	27	2	25	280	4	18
Chicken quesadilla	1 quesadilla	40	3	37	540	28	30
Chili cheese burrito	1 burrito	40	3	37	390	16	18
Cinnamon twists	1 serving	28	0	28	160	0	5
Crunchy taco, fresco	1 taco	14	2	12	150	7	7
Double Decker Taco	1 taco	39	5	34	340	14	14
Double Decker Taco Supreme	1 taco	41	5	36	380	15	18
Enchirito, beef	1 enchirito	35	5	30	380	19	18
Enchirito, beef, fresco	1 enchirito	35	5	30	270	12	9

Food	Serving size	Carbohy-drates	Fiber	Net Carbs	Calories	Protein	Fat
Enchirito, chicken	1 enchirito	33	5	28	350	23	14
Enchirito, chicken, fresco	1 enchirito	34	5	29	250	16	5
Enchirito, steak	1 enchirito	33	5	28	360	21	16
Enchirito, steak, fresco	1 enchirito	34	6	28	250	14	7
Express taco salad	1 salad	58	10	48	630	28	33
Fiesta burrito, beef	1 burrito	50	3	47	390	14	15
Fiesta burrito, chicken	1 burrito	48	3	45	370	18	12
Fiesta burrito, chicken, fresco	1 burrito	49	4	45	350	16	9
Fiesta burrito, steak	1 burrito	48	4	44	370	16	13
Fiesta taco salad	1 salad	80	12	68	870	31	47
Gordita Baja, beef	1 gordita	31	2	29	350	13	19
Gordita Baja, beef, fresco	1 gordita	31	2	29	250	12	9
Gordita Baja, chicken	1 gordita	29	2	27	320	17	15
Gordita Baja, chicken, fresco	1 gordita	29	2	27	230	15	6
Gordita Baja, steak	1 gordita	29	2	27	320	15	16
Gordita Baja, steak, fresco	1 gordita	29	3	26	230	13	7
Gordita nacho cheese, beef	1 gordita	32	2	30	300	12	13

Food	Serving size	Carbohydrates	Fiber	Net Carbs	Calories	Protein	Fat
Gordita nacho cheese, chicken	1 gordita	30	2	28	270	16	10
Gordita nacho cheese, steak	1 gordita	30	2	28	270	14	11
Gordita Supreme, beef	1 gordita	30	2	28	310	14	16
Gordita Supreme, chicken	1 gordita	28	2	26	290	17	12
Gordita Supreme, steak	1 gordita	28	2	26	290	16	13
Grande soft taco	1 taco	44	2	42	450	19	21
Grilled steak soft taco	1 taco	21	1	20	280	12	17
Grilled steak soft taco, fresco	1 taco	21	2	19	170	11	5
Grilled Stuft burrito, beef	1 burrito	79	7	72	720	27	33
Grilled Stuft burrito, chicken	1 burrito	76	7	69	680	35	26
Grilled Stuft burrito, steak	1 burrito	76	8	68	680	31	28
Mexican pizza	1 serving	47	5	42	550	21	31
Mexican rice	1 serving	23	3	20	210	6	10
MexiMelt	1 serving	23	2	21	290	15	16
Nachos	1 serving	33	2	31	320	5	19
Nachos BellGrande	1 serving	80	11	69	780	20	43
Nachos Supreme	1 serving	42	5	37	450	13	26

Food	Serving size	Carbohy- drates	Fiber	Net Carbs	Calories	Protein	Fat
Pintos, cheese	1 serving	20	6	14	180	10	7
Ranchero chicken soft taco	1 taco	21	2	19	270	14	14
Ranchero chicken soft taco, fresco	1 taco	22	2	20	170	12	4
7-Layer burrito	1 burrito	66	10	56	530	18	21
Soft taco, beef	1 taco	21	0	21	210	10	10
Soft taco, beef, fresco	1 taco	22	2	20	190	9	8
Soft Taco Supreme, beef	1 taco	23	1	22	260	11	14
Spicy chicken taco	1 taco	21	2	19	180	10	7
Spicy chicken burrito	1 burrito	50	4	46	430	14	19
Steak quesadilla	1 quesadilla	40	3	37	540	26	31
Taco	1 taco	13	0	13	170	8	10
Taco Supreme	1 taco	14	1	13	220	9	14
Tostada	1 tostada	29	7	22	250	11	10
Tostada, fresco	1 tostada	30	8	22	200	8	6

Food	Serving size	Carbohy-drates	Fiber	Net Carbs	Calories	Protein	Fat
WENDY'S							
Baked potato, bacon, cheese	10 oz.	67	7	60	560	16	25
Baked potato, broccoli, cheese	10 oz.	70	9	61	440	10	15
Baked potato, sour cream, chives	10 oz.	62	7	55	340	8	6
Barbecue sauce	1 packet	10	0	10	40	1	0
Cheeseburger, Jr.	1 serving	34	2	32	310	17	12
Cheeseburger, Jr. Bacon	1 serving	34	2	32	380	20	19
Cheeseburger, Jr. Deluxe	1 serving	36	2	34	350	18	15
Cheeseburger, Kids' Meal	1 serving	33	1	32	310	17	12
Chicken nuggets	5 pieces	13	0	13	220	10	14
Chicken sandwich, homestyle fillet	1 sandwich	57	2	55	540	29	22
Chicken sandwich, spicy fillet	1 sandwich	57	2	55	510	29	19
Chicken sandwich, Ultimate	1 sandwich	44	2	42	360	31	7
Chili	12 oz.	31	7	64	300	25	7
Dressing, Caesar	1 packet	1	0	1	150	1	16
Dressing, fat-free French	1 packet	19	0	19	80	0	0
Dressing, honey mustard	1 packet	11	0	11	280	1	26
Dressing, low-fat honey mustard	1 packet	21	0	21	110	0	3

Food	Serving size	Carbohy-drates	Fiber	Net Carbs	Calories	Protein	Fat
Dressing, oriental sesame	1 packet	19	0	19	250	1	19
Dressing, reduced-fat ranch	1 packet	6	1	5	100	1	8
Dressing, vinaigrette	1 packet	8	0	8	190	0	18
French fries, Biggie	5.6 oz.	63	7	56	440	5	19
French fries, Great Biggie	6.7 oz.	75	8	67	530	6	23
Frosty shake	16 fl. oz.	74	0	74	430	10	11
Hamburger, Big Bacon Classic	1 serving	45	3	42	580	33	29
Hamburger, Classic Single	1 serving	37	2	35	410	25	19
Hamburger, Jr.	1 serving	34	2	32	270	15	9
Hamburger, Kids' Meal	1 serving	33	1	32	270	15	9
Homestyle Chicken Strips	3 pieces	33	0	33	410	28	18
Honey mustard sauce	1 packet	6	0	6	130	0	12
Salad, chicken BLT, no dressing	1 salad	10	4	6	360	34	19
Salad, homestyle chicken strips, no dressing	1 salad	34	5	31	450	29	22
Salad, mandarin chicken, no dressing	1 salad	17	3	14	190	22	3
Salad, spring mix, no dressing	1 salad	12	5	7	180	11	11
Salad, taco supremo	1 salad	29	8	21	360	27	16
Sweet and sour sauce	1 packet	12	0	12	45	0	0

FATS, OILS, AND SPREADS

Even though fats and oils don't add any carbs to a food, you still need to be aware of them. Many prepared foods and baked goods contain unhealthy partially hydrogenated vegetable oil, or trans fats. Because these foods also tend to be high in carbs and low in nutrition, this is one type of fat to avoid. This section also includes that all-time favorite spread, mayonnaise.

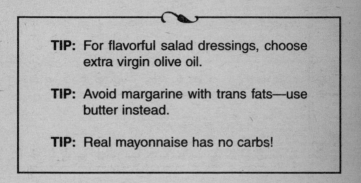

> **TIP:** For flavorful salad dressings, choose extra virgin olive oil.
>
> **TIP:** Avoid margarine with trans fats—use butter instead.
>
> **TIP:** Real mayonnaise has no carbs!

Food	Serving size	Carbohy-drates	Fiber	Net Carbs	Calories	Protein	Fat
Almond oil	1 T	0	0	0	120	0	14
Avocado oil	1 T	0	0	0	124	0	14
Beef suet	1 oz.	0	0	0	242	0	27
Butter, salted	1 T	0	0	0	102	0	12
Butter, sweet	1 T	0	0	0	102	0	12
Butter, whipped	1 T	0	0	0	67	0	8
Canola oil	1 T	0	0	0	124	0	14
Chicken fat	1 T	0	0	0	115	0	13
Coconut oil	1 T	0	0	0	117	0	14
Corn oil	1 T	0	0	0	120	0	14
Country Crock spread, soft	1 T	0	0	0	60	0	7
Country Crock spread, squeeze	1 T	0	0	0	70	0	8
Crisco	1 T	0	0	0	108	0	12
Filbert's spread, soft	1 T	0	0	0	60	0	7
Fleischmann's, soft	1 T	0	0	0	81	0	9
Fleischmann's, stick	1 T	0	0	0	99	0	11
Ghee	1 T	0	0	0	124	0	14

Food	Serving size	Carbohy-drates	Fiber	Net Carbs	Calories	Protein	Fat
Grapeseed oil	1 T	0	0	0	120	0	14
Hazelnut oil	1 T	0	0	0	120	0	14
I Can't Believe It's Not Butter, soft	1 T	0	0	0	50	0	5
I Can't Believe It's Not Butter, squeeze	1 T	0	0	0	70	0	8
Imperial, quarters	1 T	0	0	0	70	0	7
Lard	1 T	0	0	0	115	0	13
Macadamia nut oil	1 T	0	0	0	120	0	14
Margarine, corn, soft	1 t	0	0	0	34	0	4
Margarine, corn, stick	1 t	0	0	0	34	0	4
Mayonnaise, Hellman's	1 T	0	0	0	100	2	11
Mayonnaise, fat-free, Kraft	1 T	2	0	2	11	0	0
Miracle Whip	1 T	2	0	2	37	0	3
Olive oil	1 T	0	0	0	119	0	14
Palm kernel oil	1 T	0	0	0	117	0	14
Palm oil	1 T	0	0	0	120	0	14
Peanut oil	1 T	0	0	0	119	0	14
Pork fat	1 oz.	0	0	0	181	0	19

Food	Serving size	Carbohy-drates	Fiber	Net Carbs	Calories	Protein	Fat
Pork fatback	1 oz.	0	0	0	230	0	25
Promise, soft	1 T	0	0	0	80	0	8
Safflower oil	1 T	0	0	0	120	0	14
Salt pork	1 oz.	0	0	0	212	0	23
Sandwich Spred, Hellman's	1 T	2	0	2	50	0	5
Sesame oil	1 T	0	0	0	120	0	14
Shedd's, quarters	1 T	0	0	0	60	0	7
Shedd's, soft	1 T	0	0	0	100	0	11
Smart Balance Buttery	1 T	0	0	0	80	0	9
Smart Balance Light	1 T	0	0	0	45	0	5
Smart Beat squeeze	1 T	1	0	1	5	0	0
Soy oil	1 T	0	0	0	120	0	14
Sunflower oil	1 T	0	0	0	124	0	14
Vegetable oil	1 T	0	0	0	120	0	14
Walnut oil	1 T	0	0	0	120	0	14
Wheat germ oil	1 T	0	0	0	120	0	14

FISH AND SEAFOOD

In addition to being very low in carbs, fish and seafood are high in protein and contain healthy fat in the form of omega 3 fatty acids. Fish and seafood are also easy and quick to prepare and cook. To keep the carbs down, avoid breading—stick to simple baking or sautéing.

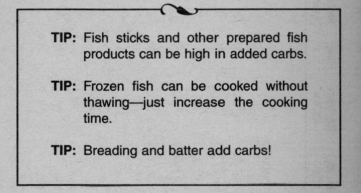

TIP: Fish sticks and other prepared fish products can be high in added carbs.

TIP: Frozen fish can be cooked without thawing—just increase the cooking time.

TIP: Breading and batter add carbs!

Food	Serving size	Carbohy-drates	Fiber	Net Carbs	Calories	Protein	Fat
(all portions are cooked)							
Anchovies, canned	5 anchovies	0	0	0	42	6	2
Bass, freshwater	3 oz.	0	0	0	124	21	4
Bass, striped	3 oz.	0	0	0	105	19	3
Bluefish	3 oz.	0	0	0	135	22	5
Carp	3 oz.	0	0	0	138	19	6
Catfish	3 oz.	0	0	0	129	16	7
Clams	3 oz.	0	0	0	126	22	2
Clams, canned	3 oz.	0	0	0	126	22	2
Cod, Atlantic	3 oz.	0	0	0	89	19	1
Cod, Pacific	3 oz.	0	0	0	89	20	1
Crab, Alaska king	3 oz.	0	0	0	82	16	1
Crab, blue	3 oz.	0	0	0	87	17	2
Crab, Dungeness	3 oz.	0	0	0	94	19	1
Crayfish	3 oz.	0	0	0	74	15	1
Eel	3 oz.	0	0	0	201	20	13
Flounder	3 oz.	0	0	0	99	21	1

Food	Serving size	Carbohy-drates	Fiber	Net Carbs	Calories	Protein	Fat
Gefilte fish	1 piece	3	0	3	35	4	1
Grouper	3 oz.	0	0	0	100	21	1
Haddock	3 oz.	0	0	0	95	21	1
Halibut	3 oz.	0	0	0	119	23	3
Herring	3 oz.	0	0	0	173	20	10
Herring, kippered	1 piece	0	0	0	87	10	5
Herring, pickled	1 piece	1	0	1	39	2	3
Lobster	3 oz.	0	0	0	83	17	1
Lox	3 oz.	0	0	0	99	16	4
Mackerel, Atlantic	3 oz.	0	0	0	223	20	15
Mackerel, jack, canned	1 cup	0	0	0	296	44	12
Mackerel, king	3 oz.	0	0	0	114	22	2
Monkfish	3 oz.	0	0	0	82	16	2
Mullet, striped	3 oz.	0	0	0	128	21	4
Mussels, blue	3 oz.	0	0	0	146	20	4
Ocean perch, Atlantic	3 oz.	0	0	0	103	20	2
Orange roughy	3 oz.	0	0	0	76	16	1

Food	Serving size	Carbohy-drates	Fiber	Net Carbs	Calories	Protein	Fat
Oysters	3 oz.	0	0	0	47	4	1
Oysters, canned	3 oz.	0	0	0	59	6	2
Perch	3 oz.	0	0	0	99	21	1
Pike, northern	3 oz.	0	0	0	96	21	1
Pike, walleye	3 oz.	0	0	0	101	21	1
Pollock, Atlantic	3 oz.	0	0	0	100	21	1
Pompano	3 oz.	0	0	0	179	20	10
Rockfish, Pacific	3 oz.	0	0	0	103	20	2
Sablefish	3 oz.	0	0	0	213	15	17
Sablefish, smoked	3 oz.	0	0	0	218	15	17
Salmon, Atlantic	3 oz.	0	0	0	175	19	11
Salmon, chinook	3 oz.	0	0	0	196	22	11
Salmon, pink, canned	3 oz.	0	0	0	118	17	5
Salmon, smoked	3 oz.	0	0	0	99	16	4
Sardines, canned, in oil	2 sardines	0	0	0	50	6	3
Scallops	3 oz.	0	0	0	75	14	1
Sea bass	3 oz.	0	0	0	105	20	3

Food	Serving size	Carbohy-drates	Fiber	Net Carbs	Calories	Protein	Fat
Sea trout	3 oz.	0	0	0	113	18	4
Shad	3 oz.	0	0	0	214	19	15
Shrimp	15 large	0	0	0	84	18	1
Smelt, rainbow	3 oz.	0	0	0	105	19	3
Snapper	3 oz.	0	0	0	109	22	2
Sole	3 oz.	0	0	0	99	21	1
Squid	3 oz.	0	0	0	109	15	4
Sturgeon	3 oz.	0	0	0	115	18	4
Sturgeon, smoked	3 oz.	0	0	0	147	27	4
Sunfish	3 oz.	0	0	0	97	21	1
Surimi	3 oz.	0	0	0	84	13	1
Swordfish	3 oz.	0	0	0	132	22	4
Tilefish	3 oz.	0	0	0	125	21	4
Trout, rainbow	3 oz.	0	0	0	144	21	6
Tuna, bluefin	3 oz.	0	0	0	156	25	5
Tuna, light, canned, oil	3 oz.	0	0	0	168	25	7
Tuna, light, canned, water	3 oz.	0	0	0	99	22	1

Food	Serving size	Carbohy-drates	Fiber	Net Carbs	Calories	Protein	Fat
Tuna, solid white, canned, oil	3 oz.	0	0	0	158	23	7
Tuna, solid white, canned, water	3 oz.	0	0	0	109	20	3
Tuna, yellowfin	3 oz.	0	0	0	118	26	1
Turbot	3 oz.	0	0	0	104	18	3
Whitefish	3 oz.	0	0	0	146	21	6
Whitefish, smoked	3 oz.	0	0	0	92	20	1

FLOUR AND BAKING PRODUCTS

One of the fun parts of following a low-carb lifestyle is learning new ways to bake using whole grains. The changes are easy to make—you'll find suggestions and great recipes in any low-carb cookbook.

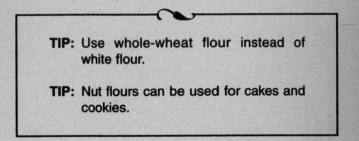

TIP: Use whole-wheat flour instead of white flour.

TIP: Nut flours can be used for cakes and cookies.

Food	Serving size	Carbohy-drates	Fiber	Net Carbs	Calories	Protein	Fat
Cornmeal, white	1 cup	94	9	85	442	10	5
Cornmeal, yellow	1 cup	94	9	85	442	9	5
Oat bran	1 cup	62	15	47	231	16	7
Pie crust, frozen	1 piecrust	64	1	63	656	6	41
Quinoa	1 cup	117	10	107	636	22	10
Rye flour, medium	1 cup	79	15	64	361	10	2
Semolina	1 cup	122	7	115	601	21	2
Soy flour, defatted	1 cup	38	18	20	329	47	1
Triticale flour	1 cup	95	19	76	439	17	2
Wheat bran	1 cup	37	25	12	125	9	3
Wheat flour, all-purpose, white, enriched	1 cup	95	3	92	455	13	1
Wheat flour, whole wheat	1 cup	87	15	72	407	16	2
Wheat germ, toasted	1 cup	56	15	41	432	33	12

Food	Serving size	Carbohy-drates	Fiber	Net Carbs	Calories	Protein	Fat
REDUCED-CARB PRODUCTS							
All-purpose batter mix, Atkins	2 t	5	4	1	30	3	0
Bake mix, Atkins	1 cup	32	20	12	320	52	2
Bake mix, Carbquick	1 oz.	9	7	2	50	3	4
Bake mix, Low Carb Chef's	1 T	4	1	3	45	6	3
Bake mix, Zero Carb	1 oz.	4	4	0	110	22	1
Flour replacement blend, Low Carb Chef's	¼ cup	15	9	6	70	9	0
French crepe mix, Atkins	1 crepe	2	2	0	12	2	0
Piecrust mix, Atkins	1 piecrust	28	21	3	126	28	0
Piecrust mix, MiniCarb	1 piecrust	6	0	6	105	9	7
ThickenThin Not/Starch thickener, Atkins	1 t	2	2	0	7	0	0
Thick It Up	½ t	1	1	0	6	0	0

FROZEN BREAKFASTS

Studies have shown that people who regularly eat a nutritious breakfast have an easier time controlling their weight—and that skipping breakfast is a good way to sabotage weight-loss efforts. Frozen breakfasts make it easier to have a good breakfast even on a busy morning, but be selective. Many of these products are high in carbs.

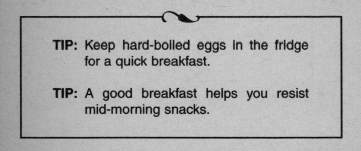

TIP: Keep hard-boiled eggs in the fridge for a quick breakfast.

TIP: A good breakfast helps you resist mid-morning snacks.

Food	Serving size	Carbohy-drates	Fiber	Net Carbs	Calories	Protein	Fat
Breakfast burrito	1 burrito	28	1	27	212	10	7
Egg, Canadian bacon, cheese, muffin, Swanson	1 package	25	2	23	290	14	15
El Monterey Supreme Burrito, egg, sausage	1 burrito	34	1	33	293	19	13
French toast sticks, syrup, Swanson	1 package	50	2	48	320	7	10
Hot Pockets, bacon, egg, cheese	1 pocket	20	1	19	167	6	7
Hot pockets, ham, egg, cheese	1 pocket	17	1	16	155	6	7
Hot Pockets, sausage, egg, cheese	1 pocket	19	1	18	163	6	7
Jimmy Dean Breakfast Sandwich, bacon, egg, cheese, biscuit	1 sandwich	26	0	26	290	13	15
Jimmy Dean Breakfast Sandwich, sausage biscuit	1 sandwich	23	1	22	385	10	28
Jimmy Dean Breakfast Sandwich, sausage, egg, cheese biscuit	1 sandwich	27	0	27	380	14	24
Jimmy Dean Breakfast Sandwich, sausage, egg, cheese muffin	1 sandwich	26	0	26	380	13	25
Lean Pockets, bacon, egg, cheese	1 pocket	21	2	19	153	7	5

Food	Serving size	Carbohy-drates	Fiber	Net Carbs	Calories	Protein	Fat
Lean Pockets, sausage, egg, cheese	1 pocket	19	2	17	145	7	5
Low-fat eggs, pancakes, Swanson	1 entrée	30	0	30	220	10	7
Scrambled eggs, burrito, Swanson	1 entrée	25	0	25	200	7	8
Scrambled eggs, sausage, potatoes	6 oz. entrée	17	1	16	361	13	27
Scrambled eggs, sausage, potatoes, Swanson	6 oz. entrée	21	3	18	360	12	26
Toaster Scrambles pastry, bacon and sausage	1 entrée	14	0	14	180	4	12
Toaster Scrambles pastry, cheese, egg, ham	1 entrée	14	0	14	180	4	12
Toaster Scrambles pastry, cheese, egg, sausage	1 entrée	14	0	14	180	4	12
Toaster Scrambles pastry, western	1 entrée	14	0	14	170	4	11

FROZEN MEALS AND ENTREES

For convenience and variety, it's hard to beat frozen meals. The good features of frozen meals can be offset, however, by high carb counts. Skip the fried foods and pasta choices and go for the products that come with vegetables and smaller portions of high-carb foods such as mashed potatoes or noodles. Remember to check the food facts label to make sure you're not getting more carbs than you realize.

TIP: Entrees such as fried chicken are high in carbs.

TIP: Have a salad with your frozen meal for extra nutrition.

TIP: Frozen meals can help you control portions.

TIP: Most frozen meals are ready in under 10 minutes.

Food	Serving size	Carbohy-drates	Fiber	Net Carbs	Calories	Protein	Fat
Beef, broccoli stir fry, Green Giant	10 oz. meal	15	4	11	290	27	13
Beef macaroni, Healthy Choice	8.5 oz. entrée	34	5	29	211	14	2
Beef patty, vegetables, Banquet	9.5 oz. meal	22	2	20	310	11	20
Beef pepper steak oriental, Healthy Choice	9.5 oz. entrée	34	2	32	260	19	5
Beef pot roast, Marie Callender's	15 oz. meal	55	3	52	500	23	17
Beef pot roast, Healthy Choice	11 oz. meal	41	8	33	300	20	6
Beef pot roast, whipped potatoes, Stouffers Lean Cuisine	9 oz. entrée	22	4	18	207	17	5
Beef stew, Green Giant	10 oz.	27	4	23	180	11	4
Beef stew, hearty, Banquet	8.7 oz. entrée	18	4	14	170	10	7
Beef stroganoff, Healthy Choice	11 oz. meal	40	7	33	320	22	8
Beef stroganoff, Marie Callender's	13 oz. meal	59	4	55	600	30	27
Beef tips francais, Healthy Choice	9.5 oz. entrée	40	4	36	300	20	7
Burrito, bean and cheese, Patio	1 burrito	46	4	42	300	9	9
Burrito, chicken, Patio	1 burrito	44	2	42	290	11	8
Chicken alfredo, Green Giant	8 oz.	37	2	25	270	15	7
Chicken bbq, vegetables, Weight Watchers	7.4 oz. entrée	26	1	25	217	19	4

Food	Serving size	Carbohy-drates	Fiber	Net Carbs	Calories	Protein	Fat
Chicken, broccoli alfredo, Banquet	6.8 oz. entrée	28	3	25	270	11	12
Chicken, broccoli alfredo, Healthy Choice	11.5 oz. meal	34	2	32	300	25	7
Chicken cacciatore, pasta, vegetable, Healthy Choice	12.5 oz. meal	36	5	31	266	22	4
Chicken Cantonese, Healthy Choice	10.8 oz. meal	34	2	32	280	22	6
Chicken, cheesy pasta, Green Giant	8 oz.	39	3	36	270	13	7
Chicken cordon bleu, Marie Callender's	13 oz. meal	58	6	52	610	33	28
Chicken, country fried, Marie Callender's	16 oz. meal	63	6	57	620	24	30
Chicken, country herb, Healthy Choice	12 oz. meal	44	3	41	320	18	8
Chicken, dumplings, Marie Callender's	14 oz. meal	34	4	30	390	17	20
Chicken fiesta, Healthy Choice Bowl	9.5 oz. bowl	34	3	31	220	15	2
Chicken fingers, Banquet	7.1 oz. meal	67	6	61	740	22	43
Chicken, fried, Banquet	9 oz. meal	35	2	33	470	21	27
Chicken, fried, Morton	9 oz. meal	30	3	27	470	20	30
Chicken, fried, boneless, Banquet	8 oz. meal	41	3	38	540	16	34
Chicken, garlic lemon, Health Choice Bowl	9.5 oz. bowl	48	4	44	300	18	4

Food	Serving size	Carbohy-drates	Fiber	Net Carbs	Calories	Protein	Fat
Chicken, garlic sauce, pasta, vegetable, Tyson	9 oz. entrée	22	4	18	214	17	7
Chicken, honey glazed, Healthy Choice	10 oz. meal	32	4	28	270	21	7
Chicken, noodles, Green Giant	8 oz.	45	3	42	290	14	6
Chicken, noodles, Marie Callender's	13 oz. meal	42	5	38	520	21	30
Chicken, noodles, Stouffer's	10 oz. entrée	31	1	30	419	17	25
Chicken nuggets, Banquet	6.7 oz. meal	42	4	38	430	14	23
Chicken nuggets, Morton	7 oz. meal	31	2	29	340	12	19
Chicken parmigiana, Healthy Choice	11.5 oz. meal	46	3	43	330	19	8
Chicken parmigiana, Marie Callender's	16 oz. meal	63	5	58	660	30	32
Chicken piccata, rice, vegetable, Smart Ones	9 oz. entrée	36	2	34	250	15	5
Chicken pie, hearty, Banquet	8 oz. entrée	39	2	37	460	11	29
Chicken, vegetables marsala, Healthy Choice	11.5 oz. entrée	32	3	29	240	20	4
Chimichanga, Banquet	9.5 oz. meal	56	9	47	500	13	24
Egg rolls, chicken, Chun King	6 mini rolls	25	2	23	210	6	9

Food	Serving size	Carbohy-drates	Fiber	Net Carbs	Calories	Protein	Fat
Egg rolls, chicken, LaChoy	6 mini rolls	25	2	23	210	6	9
Egg rolls, shrimp, Chun King	6 mini rolls	28	2	26	190	5	6
Egg rolls, shrimp, LaChoy	6 mini rolls	28	2	26	190	5	6
Enchiladas, beef, Banquet	11 oz. meal	54	8	46	370	10	12
Enchiladas, beef, Patio	2 pieces	29	5	24	210	5	8
Enchiladas, cheese, Banquet	11 oz. meal	56	8	48	360	12	10
Enchiladas, suiza, Healthy Choice	10 oz. entrée	43	5	38	280	14	6
Fettuccini alfredo, Healthy Choice	8 oz. entrée	36	4	32	240	10	6
Fish, herb baked, Healthy Choice	10.9 oz. meal	54	5	49	340	16	7
Fish, lemon pepper, Healthy Choice	10.7 oz. meal	50	5	45	320	14	7
Fish sticks, Banquet	6.6 oz. meal	33	4	29	290	11	13
Garlic chicken pasta, Green Giant	8 oz. serving	30	3	27	250	3	7
Lasagna, Banquet	8 oz. entrée	33	2	31	270	14	10
Lasagna, Marie Callender's	8.9 oz. entrée	35	3	32	350	15	17
Macaroni and cheese, Banquet	12 oz. meal	57	5	52	420	15	14
Macaroni and cheese, Healthy Choice	9 oz. entrée	40	3	37	270	13	6
Macaroni and cheese, Marie Callender's	12 oz. meal	55	5	50	540	25	24

Food	Serving size	Carbohy-drates	Fiber	Net Carbs	Calories	Protein	Fat
Meatloaf, mashed potatoes, Banquet	9.5 oz. meal	23	3	20	280	12	16
Pocket sandwich, beef, cheddar, Hot Pockets	5 oz. pocket	39	0	39	403	16	20
Pocket sandwich, broccoli, cheddar, Weight Watchers	5 oz. pocket	40	0	40	266	13	6
Pocket sandwich, Chicken, Lean Pockets	4.5 oz. pocket	43	0	34	233	10	6
Pork chop, country fried, Marie Callender's	15 oz. meal	50	8	42	540	23	28
Pork rib, Banquet	10 oz. meal	40	4	36	400	17	19
Pot pie, beef, Banquet	7 oz. pie	38	1	37	400	9	23
Pot pie, chicken, Banquet	7 oz. pie	36	1	35	382	10	22
Pot pie, chicken, Stouffer's	10 oz. pie	37	3	34	572	23	37
Salisbury steak, Marie Callender's	14 oz. meal	51	6	45	550	30	25
Salisbury steak, potato, corn, green beans, Stouffer's	16 oz. meal	49	5	44	550	28	27
Swedish meatballs, pasta, Stouffer's Lean Cuisine	9 oz. entrée	31	3	28	276	22	7
Sweet and sour chicken, Healthy Choice	11 oz. meal	53	5	48	360	20	7

Food	Serving size	Carbohy-drates	Fiber	Net Carbs	Calories	Protein	Fat
Sweet and sour chicken, Marie Callender's	14 oz. meal	86	7	79	570	23	15
Tuna noodle casserole, Stouffer's	10 oz. entrée	36	2	34	360	18	16
Turkey, mashed potatoes, Smart Ones	10 oz. entrée	39	4	35	240	16	4
Turkey breast, Healthy Choice	10.5 oz. meal	40	5	35	290	22	5
Veal parmigiana, Banquet	9 oz. meal	30	4	26	290	8	15

FRUIT

Of all the popular misconceptions about low-carb dieting, not eating fruit probably tops the list. Yes, you *can* enjoy fruit on your low-carb diet! In fact, it's encouraged—in moderation. Almost all fruits are good, low-glycemic carbs, packed with fiber, vitamins, minerals, and other nutritional benefits. And with the exception of avocados, fruits have little or no dietary fat.

Choose the most colorful, low-carb fruits possible. Berries are an especially good choice—they're low in carbs, high in flavor, and rich in nutrition.

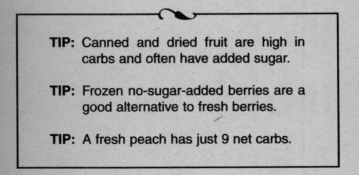

TIP: Canned and dried fruit are high in carbs and often have added sugar.

TIP: Frozen no-sugar-added berries are a good alternative to fresh berries.

TIP: A fresh peach has just 9 net carbs.

Food	Serving size	Carbohy-drates	Fiber	Net Carbs	Calories	Protein	Fat
Apple, raw	1 med.	21	4	17	81	0	0
Applesauce, sweetened	1 cup	51	3	48	194	0	0
Apricots, canned, heavy syrup	1 cup'	55	4	51	214	1	0
Apricots, dried	1 cup	81	10	71	313	4	1
Apricots, raw	4 med.	17	4	13	74	2	0
Avocado, California, raw	½ med.	6	4	2	153	2	15
Avocado, Florida, raw	½ med.	16	8	8	170	2.5	16
Banana chips	1 oz.	17	2	15	147	1	10
Banana, raw	1 med.	27	3	25	105	1	0
Blackberries, canned, heavy syrup	1 cup	59	9	50	236	3	0
Blackberries, frozen, unsweetened	1 cup	24	8	16	97	1	2
Blackberries, raw	1 cup	18	4	17	74	1	0.5
Blueberries, frozen, sweetened	1 cup	51	5	46	186	1	0
Blueberries, raw	1 cup	21	4	17	81	1	0
Boysenberries, canned, heavy syrup	1 cup	57	7	50	225	3	0
Cantaloupe, raw	1 cup	15	1	14	56	1	0
Carambola (star fruit), raw	1 med.	7	3	4	30	0	0

Food	Serving size	Carbohy-drates	Fiber	Net Carbs	Calories	Protein	Fat
Casaba melon, raw	1 cup	11	1	10	44	1.5	0
Cherries, sour, canned, syrup	1 cup	60	3	57	233	2	0
Cherries, sweet, frozen, sweetened	1 cup	58	5	53	231	1	0
Cherries, sweet, raw	10	19	3	16	84	1	1
Cranberries, raw	1 cup	12	4	8	47	0	0
Cranberry sauce, jellied	½" slice	22	1	21	86	0	0
Dates, dried	1	6	1	5	23	0	0
Figs, canned, syrup	1	6	1	5	25	0	0
Figs, dried	1	12	2	10	48	1	0
Figs, raw	1 med.	10	2	8	37	0	0
Fruit cocktail, canned, heavy syrup	1 cup	47	3	44	181	0	0
Fruit salad, canned, heavy syrup	1 cup	49	3	45	186	0	0
Grapefruit, canned, heavy syrup	1 cup	39	1	38	152	0	0
Grapefruit, raw, pink/red/white	½ med.	9	1	8	37	1	0
Grapes, green/red	1 cup	28	2	26	114	1	0
Guava, raw	1 med.	11	5	6	46	1	0
Honeydew melon, raw	1 cup	16	1	15	62	1	0

Food	Serving size	Carbohy-drates	Fiber	Net Carbs	Calories	Protein	Fat
Kiwifruit, raw	1 med.	11	3	8	46	1	0
Lemon, raw	1 med.	5	2	3	17	1	0
Lime, raw	1 med.	7	2	5	20	0	0
Mandarin oranges, canned, syrup	1 cup	24	2	22	92	0	0
Mango, raw	1 med.	35	4	31	135	1	1
Nectarine, raw	1 med.	16	2	14	67	1	0
Orange, navel, raw	1 med.	16	3	13	64	1	0
Papaya, raw	1 med.	30	6	24	119	2	0
Passion fruit, raw	1 med.	4	2	2	17	0	0
Peach, canned, heavy syrup	1 cup	52	3	49	194	1	0
Peach, raw	1 med.	11	2	9	37	0	0
Pear, canned, heavy syrup	1 cup	51	4	47	197	0	0
Pear, raw	1 med.	25	4	21	98	0	0
Persimmon, raw	1 med.	31	6	25	118	0	0
Pineapple, canned, heavy syrup	1 cup	51	2	49	199	1	0
Pineapple, raw	1 cup	19	2	17	76	0	1
Plums, canned, heavy syrup	1	11	1	10	41	0	0

Food	Serving size	Carbohy-drates	Fiber	Net Carbs	Calories	Protein	Fat
Plum, raw	1 med.	9	1	7	36	0	0
Pomegranate, raw	1 med.	26	1	25	105	1.5	0
Prunes, canned, heavy syrup	5	24	3	21	90	1	0
Prune, dried	1	5	1	4	20	0	0
Raisins, golden	1 cup	115	6	109	438	5	0
Raisins, dark	1 cup	124	8	116	520	4	0
Raspberries, frozen, sweetened	1 cup	60	8	52	233	2	0
Raspberries, raw	1 cup	14	8	6	60	1	1
Strawberries, frozen, sweetened	1 cup	54	5	49	199	1	0
Strawberries, raw	1 cup	10	3	7	43	1	0
Tangerine, raw	1 med.	9	2	7	37	0	0
Watermelon, raw	1 cup	11	1	10	49	1	0

ICE CREAM AND FROZEN DESSERTS

Life without ice cream is inconceivable, which is why you can still have it even when you follow a reduced-carb lifestyle. Amazingly, premium ice cream and low-fat ice cream have about the same number of carbs—in fact, sometimes low-fat ice cream has *more* carbs. If you really need to watch your carbs, choose a reduced-carb, not on a reduced-fat, ice cream.

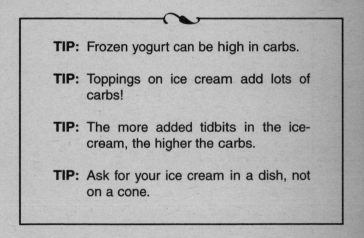

TIP: Frozen yogurt can be high in carbs.

TIP: Toppings on ice cream add lots of carbs!

TIP: The more added tidbits in the ice-cream, the higher the carbs.

TIP: Ask for your ice cream in a dish, not on a cone.

Food	Serving size	Carbohy-drates	Fiber	Net Carbs	Calories	Protein	Fat
Baskin-Robbins, Berries 'n Banana, low-fat	½ cup	25	1	24	138	5	2
Baskin-Robbins, chocolate	½ cup	33	0	33	278	5	14
Baskin-Robbins, chocolate chip	½ cup	28	1	27	276	5	16
Baskin-Robbins, chocolate chip, low-fat	½ cup	30	1	29	177	4	5
Baskin-Robbins, Espresso 'n Cream, low-fat	½ cup	32	1	31	184	5	4
Baskin-Robbins, pineapple coconut, low-fat	½ cup	27	0	27	142	4	2
Baskin-Robbins, Rocky Road	½ cup	36	1	35	299	5	15
Baskin-Robbins vanilla	½ cup	26	0	26	264	4	16
Ben & Jerry's, Cherry Garcia	½ cup	26	1	25	255	4	15
Ben & Jerry's, Chunky Monkey	½ cup	30	1	29	307	4	19
Ben & Jerry's, coffee	½ cup	21	0	21	235	4	15
Ben & Jerry's, mocha latte, low-fat	½ cup	28	0	28	150	5	2
Ben & Jerry's, New York Super Fudge, no sugar added	½ cup	18	5	13	250	4	18
Ben & Jerry's, peanut butter cup	½ cup	29	2	17	382	8	26

Food	Serving size	Carbohy-drates	Fiber	Net Carbs	Calories	Protein	Fat
Ben & Jerry's, S'mores	½ cup	34	1	33	260	3	12
Ben & Jerry's, S'mores, low-fat	½ cup	35	1	34	190	5	2
Ben & Jerry's, strawberry	½ cup	26	0	26	246	4	14
Ben & Jerry's, vanilla	½ cup	21	0	21	244	4	16
Ben & Jerry's, Wavy Gravy	½ cup	32	9	23	340	7	20
Breyer's, butter pecan	½ cup	14	0	14	167	3	11
Breyer's, butter pecan, no sugar added	½ cup	15	0	15	135	3	7
Breyer's, chocolate	½ cup	17	1	16	152	3	8
Breyer's, chocolate, 98% fat-free no sugar added	½ cup	21	4	17	110	3	2
Breyer's, chocolate caramel,	½ cup	18	0	18	162	3	4
Breyer's, chocolate chip	½ cup	17	0	17	157	2	9
Breyer's, deep chocolate fudge	½ cup	21	1	20	204	2	12
Breyer's, light vanilla	½ cup	18	0	18	125	3	5
Breyer's, vanilla	½ cup	15	0	15	113	3	5
Breyer's, vanilla, 98% fat free	½ cup	21	4	17	106	2	2
Breyer's, vanilla fudge twirl, no sugar added	½ cup	19	0	19	124	3	4

Food	Serving size	Carbohy-drates	Fiber	Net Carbs	Calories	Protein	Fat
Carvel, chocolate	½ cup	22	0	22	194	4	10
Carvel, chocolate, no fat	½ cup	28	0	28	120	2	0
Carvel, chocolate, soft serve	½ cup	22	0	22	195	4	10
Carvel, chocolate, soft serve, no fat	½ cup	28	0	28	120	2	0
Carvel, vanilla	½ cup	21	0	21	194	5	10
Carvel, vanilla, no fat	½ cup	25	0	25	116	4	0
Carvel, vanilla, no sugar added	½ cup	25	0	25	147	5	3
Carvel, vanilla, soft serve	½ cup	21	0	21	195	5	10
Carvel, vanilla, soft serve, no fat	½ cup	25	0	25	115	4	0
Dove, chocolate	1 bar	34	3	31	341	4	21
Dove, vanilla	1 bar	33	1	32	337	4	21
Edy's, almond praline	½ cup	21	0	21	168	3	8
Edy's, chocolate fudge, fat free	½ cup	26	0	26	120	3	0
Edy's, cookie dough	½ cup	21	0	21	177	3	9
Edy's, French vanilla	½ cup	17	0	17	160	2	9
Edy's, mocha fudge, no sugar added	½ cup	13	0	13	90	3	3
Edy's, triple chocolate, no sugar added	½ cup	13	0	13	100	3	4
Edy's, Turtle Sundae	½ cup	18	0	18	165	3	9

Food	Serving size	Carbohy-drates	Fiber	Net Carbs	Calories	Protein	Fat
Frozen yogurt, chocolate	½ cup	22	0	22	140	3	5
Frozen yogurt, chocolate, soft serve	½ cup	18	0	18	115	3	4
Frozen yogurt, strawberry	½ cup	22	0	22	140	3	5
Frozen yogurt, vanilla	½ cup	22	0	22	140	3	5
Frozen yogurt, vanilla, soft serve	½ cup	17	0	17	114	3	4
FrozFruit, cherry	1 bar	16	1	15	68	1	0
FrozFruit, lemon	1 bar	19	0	19	76	0	0
FrozFruit, strawberry	1 bar	23	1	22	92	0	0
FrozFruit, tropical	1 bar	21	1	20	89	0	0
Fudgsicle	1 bar	18	0	18	98	3	2
Haagen-Dazs, butter pecan	½ cup	21	1	20	311	5	23
Haagen-Dazs, Cookies & Cream	½ cup	23	0	23	265	5	17
Haagen-Dazs, mint chip	½ cup	26	1	25	295	5	19
Haagen-Dazs, rum raisin	½ cup	22	0	22	257	4	17
Italian ices	½ cup	16	0	16	61	0	0
Klondike	1 bar	24	0	24	279	3	19
Popsicle	1 bar	11	0	11	42	0	0
Sorbet, Edy's	½ cup	33	0	33	131	0	0

Food	Serving size	Carbohy-drates	Fiber	Net Carbs	Sugar Alcohol	Calories	Protein	Fat
REDUCED-CARB PRODUCTS								
Atkins, frozen fudge bar mix	2 bars	4	4	0	0	22	2	0
CarbSmart, fudge	½ cup	11	1	0	10	128	2	8
CarbSmart, ice cream sandwich	1 bar	10	1	0	9	84	2	4
CarbSmart, vanilla	½ cup	10	3	0	7	150	2	9
Endulge, butter pecan	½ cup	12	4	4	4	170	2	15
Endulge, chocolate	½ cup	13	5	4	4	140	2	12
Endulge, chocolate fudge bars	1 bar	12	5	4	3	130	2	11
Endulge, chocolate fudge swirl bars	1 bar	12	5	4	3	180	3	16
Endulge, peanut butter swirl bars	1 bar	12	4	4	4	180	2	17
Endulge, vanilla	½ cup	13	4	5	4	140	2	12
Endulge, vanilla fudge swirl	½ cup	14	4	6	4	140	2	10
Endulge, vanilla fudge swirl bars	1 bar	12	4	4	4	180	2	16
Pierre's Carb Success, chocolate	½ cup	13	6	4	3	120	3	9
Pierre's Carb Success, vanilla	½ cup	13	6	4	3	120	3	9

JAM, JELLY, SUGAR, AND SYRUPS

Here's a category of food where carbs can start to creep in. It's all too easy to reduce carbs by cutting back on bread, for instance, and then pile on enough jelly to add back all the carbs! Go easy on the jams, jellies, syrups, and other sweeteners. There are now many brands that have no added sugar or are sugar-free. And remember, a little sweetness can go a long way.

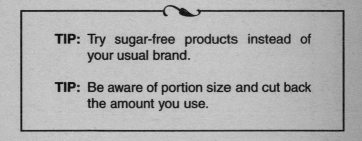

TIP: Try sugar-free products instead of your usual brand.

TIP: Be aware of portion size and cut back the amount you use.

Food	Serving size	Carbohy-drates	Fiber	Net Carbs	Calories	Protein	Fat
Apple butter	1 T	7	0	7	29	0	0
Honey	1 T	17	0	17	64	0	0
Jam	1 T	14	0	14	56	0	0
Jam, 100% fruit, Smucker's	1 T	10	0	10	44	0	0
Jam, sugar-free, Smucker's	1 T	5	0	5	20	0	0
Jam, strawberry, Dickinson's	1 T	13	0	13	52	0	0
Jam, strawberry, all-fruit, Polaner	1 T	10	0	10	42	0	0
Jelly	1 T	13	0	13	54	0	0
Marmalade, orange	1 T	13	0	13	49	0	0
Molasses	1 T	14	0	14	53	0	0
Preserves	1 T	14	0	14	56	0	0
Sugar, brown	1 T	9	0	9	34	0	0
Sugar, brown	1 cup	141	0	141	545	0	0
Sugar, powdered	1 T	8	0	8	31	0	0
Sugar, white	1 t	4	0	4	16	0	0
Sugar, white	1 T	12	0	12	48	0	0

Food	Serving size	Carbohy-drates	Fiber	Net Carbs	Calories	Protein	Fat
Syrup, corn, light	1 T	15	0	15	56	0	0
Syrup, maple	1 T	13	0	13	52	0	0
Syrup, pancake	1 T	15	0	15	57	0	0
Syrup, pancake, reduced calorie	1 T	7	0	7	25	0	0

MILK AND MILK BEVERAGES

Although milk is relatively high in carbohydrates from the lactose, or milk sugar, it contains, you can still use it. Stick to small portions, however, or choose a reduced-carb product. The amount of fat in milk doesn't affect the carbs—nonfat milk has the same amount of carbs as whole milk.

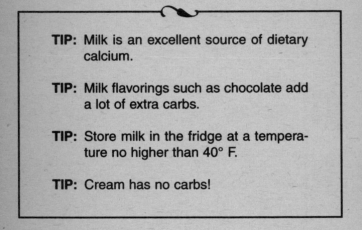

TIP: Milk is an excellent source of dietary calcium.

TIP: Milk flavorings such as chocolate add a lot of extra carbs.

TIP: Store milk in the fridge at a temperature no higher than 40° F.

TIP: Cream has no carbs!

MILK AND CREAM

Food	Serving size	Carbohy-drates	Fiber	Net Carbs	Calories	Protein	Fat
Buttermilk, cultured	8 fl. oz.	12	0	12	98	8	2
Chocolate, lowfat milk	8 fl. oz.	26	0	26	158	8	3
Chocolate, 2% milk	8 fl. oz.	26	0	26	180	8	5
Chocolate, whole milk	8 fl. oz.	26	0	26	208	8	9
Condensed, sweetened, canned	1 fl. oz.	21	0	21	123	3	3
Cream, light	1 T	0	0	0	29	0	3
Cream, heavy	1 T	0	0	0	52	0	6
Eggnog, nonalcoholic	8 fl. oz.	34	0	34	343	10	19
Evaporated, whole, canned	1 fl. oz.	3	0	3	42	2	2
Half & half	1 T	1	0	1	20	0	2
Lactaid, calcium added	8 fl. oz.	13	0	13	80	8	0
Lactaid, fat-free	8 fl. oz.	13	0	13	80	8	0
Lactaid, lowfat	8 fl. oz.	13	0	13	110	8	3
Lactaid, 2% fat	8 fl. oz.	12	0	12	130	8	5
Lactaid, whole	8 fl. oz.	12	0	12	150	8	8
Lowfat, 1% fat	8 fl. oz.	12	0	12	102	8	3

Food	Serving size	Carbohy-drates	Fiber	Net Carbs	Calories	Protein	Fat
Malted milk, whole milk	8 fl. oz.	28	0	28	239	10	10
Nonfat milk	8 fl. oz.	12	0	12	86	8	0
Reduced fat, 2% fat	8 fl. oz.	12	0	12	122	8	5
Sour cream	1 T	0	0	0	26	0	3
Sour cream, fat-free	1 T	5	0	5	29	2	0
Sour cream, reduced-fat	1 T	1	0	1	47	1	4
Whole milk	8 fl. oz.	12	0	12	149	8	8
NONDAIRY MILKS							
Almond milk, chocolate	8 fl. oz.	22	1	21	110	1	3
Almond milk, vanilla	8 fl. oz.	16	0	16	90	1	3
Creamer	1 T	2	0	2	20	0	2
Rice beverage, Rice Dream	8 fl. oz.	25	0	25	120	0	2
Rice beverage, Westbrae	8 fl. oz.	20	0	20	110	1	3
Rice beverage, vanilla, Westbrae	8 fl. oz.	20	0	20	110	1	3
Vitamite 100 nondairy beverage	8 fl. oz.	14	0	14	110	3	5

REDUCED-CARB PRODUCTS

Food	Serving size	Carbohy-drates	Fiber	Net Carbs	Calories	Protein	Fat
Carb Countdown, dairy beverage	8 fl. oz.	3	0	3	130	12	8
Carb Countdown, fat-free dairy beverage	8 fl. oz.	3	0	3	70	12	0
Carb Countdown, 2% dairy beverage	8 fl. oz.	3	0	3	100	12	5
Carb Countdown, 2% chocolate dairy beverage	8 fl. oz.	3	1	2	100	12	5

NUTS AND SEEDS

A favorite snack food for low-carb dieters, nuts are low in net carbs and high in protein. They are also high in good fats, including monounsaturated fat. Several studies have shown that eating just an ounce of nuts a day can help reduce your risk of heart disease. The benefit is believed to come from the healthy fat in the nuts.

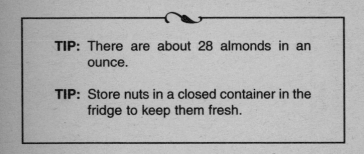

TIP: There are about 28 almonds in an ounce.

TIP: Store nuts in a closed container in the fridge to keep them fresh.

Food	Serving size	Carbohy-drates	Fiber	Net Carbs	Calories	Protein	Fat
Almond butter	1 T	3	1	2	101	2	10
Almonds, dry roasted	1 oz.	6	3	3	169	6	15
Almonds, honey roasted	1 oz.	8	4	4	169	5	14
Cashew butter	1 T	4	0	4	94	3	8
Cashews, dry roasted	1 oz.	9	1	8	163	4	13
Cashews, honey roasted	1 oz.	7	1	6	150	4	13
Chestnuts, roasted	1 oz.	15	1	14	69	1	1
Coconut, dried, sweetened, flaked	1 oz.	14	1	13	134	1	9
Corn nuts	1 oz.	21	2	19	124	2	4
Hazelnuts (filberts), dry roasted	1 oz.	5	3	2	183	4	17
Macadamia nuts, dry roasted	1 oz.	4	2	2	200	2	22
Mixed nuts, dry roasted	1 oz.	7	3	4	168	5	15
Mixed nuts, oil roasted	1 oz.	6	3	3	175	5	16
Peanut butter, chunky	2 T	7	2	5	188	8	16
Peanut butter, chunky, Carb Options	2 T	5	2	3	190	7	17
Peanut butter, smooth	2 T	6	2	4	190	8	16
Peanut butter, smooth, Carb Options	2 T	5	2	3	190	7	17

Food	Serving size	Carbohy-drates	Fiber	Net Carbs	Calories	Protein	Fat
Peanuts, dry roasted	1 oz.	6	2	4	166	7	14
Peanuts, honey roasted	1 oz.	10	2	8	150	6	11
Peanuts, oil roasted	1 oz.	5	2	3	165	8	14
Pecans, dry roasted	1 oz.	4	3	1	201	3	21
Pecans, oil roasted	1 oz.	4	3	1	203	3	21
Pine nuts	1 oz.	4	1	3	160	7	14
Pistachios, dry roasted	1 oz.	8	3	5	162	6	13
Pumpkin seeds, roasted	1 oz.	4	1	3	148	9	12
Soy nut butter	2 T	10	1	9	170	8	11
Soy nut butter, Beanit	2 T	5	5	0	170	10	12
Soy nuts, dry roasted	1 oz.	7	2	5	97	9	5
Sunflower seeds, dry roasted	1 oz.	7	3	4	165	6	14
Sunflower seeds, oil roasted	1 oz.	4	2	2	174	6	16
Tahini (sesame butter)	1 T	3	1	2	89	3	8
Walnuts	1 oz.	4	2	2	185	4	19

PASTA

Few foods are as inexpensive, versatile, and delicious as pasta. While pasta is generally high in carbs, you can still find ways to enjoy it. If you're past the stage of watching every net carb gram, you can enjoy pasta now and then in small portions. No matter how closely you're watching the carbs, you can cut the net carbs down by selecting whole wheat pasta or soy-based pasta instead of durum wheat or semolina versions. You can also try some of the new reduced-carb pasta products.

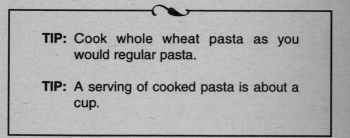

TIP: Cook whole wheat pasta as you would regular pasta.

TIP: A serving of cooked pasta is about a cup.

(all portions are cooked)

Food	Serving size	Carbohydrates	Fiber	Net Carbs	Calories	Protein	Fat
Corn pasta	1 cup	39	7	32	176	4	1
Egg noodles	1 cup	40	2	38	213	8	2
Elbows	1 cup	40	2	38	210	8	2
Elbows, soy, Soy 7	1 cup	33	2	31	200	13	1
Linguini	1 cup	40	2	38	210	8	2
Linguini, soy, Soy 7	1 cup	33	2	31	200	13	1
Lo mein, chicken, Green Giant	8 oz.	30	3	27	250	16	7
Macaroni	1 cup	40	2	38	197	7	1
Macaroni, whole wheat	1 cup	37	4	33	174	8	1
Noodles, whole wheat, Ronzoni	1 cup	41	6	35	180	7	1
Penne	1 cup	40	2	38	210	8	2
Penne, soy, Soy 7	1 cup	33	2	31	200	13	1
Ramen noodles	1 cup	37	0	37	296	6	14
Rice noodles	1 cup	44	2	42	192	2	0
Rotelle, vegetables, herbed butter sauce, Birds Eye	1 cup	26	1	25	160	5	4

Food	Serving size	Carbohydrates	Fiber	Net Carbs	Calories	Protein	Fat
Shells, whole wheat, Hodgson Mill	1 cup	34	6	28	190	9	1
Soba Japanese noodles	1 cup	24	1	23	113	6	0
Somen Japanese noodles	1 cup	49	1	48	231	7	0
Spaghetti	1 cup	40	2	38	197	7	1
Spaghetti, soy, Soy 7	1 cup	33	2	31	200	13	1
Spaghetti, spinach	1 cup	37	1	36	182	6	1
Spaghetti, spinach, Westbrae	1 cup	38	8	30	180	9	2
Spaghetti, whole wheat	1 cup	37	6	31	174	8	1
Spaghetti, whole wheat, Hodgson Mill	1 cup	40	6	34	190	9	1
Spaghetti, whole wheat, Westbrae	1 cup	39	9	30	200	9	2
Tortellini, cheese, spinach, Barilla	1 cup	32	3	29	230	8	7
Tortellini, three-cheese, Barilla	1 cup	33	3	30	230	8	8
Vegetables, shell, garlic butter sauce, Birds Eye	1 package	32	3	29	270	6	13

Food	Serving size	Carbohy-drates	Fiber	Net Carbs	Calories	Protein	Fat
REDUCED-CARB PRODUCTS							
Elbows, Carb Fit	1 cup	16	7	9	200	25	4
Elbows, Dreamfields	1 cup	42	37	5	190	7	1
Elbows, Mueller's	1 cup	31	12	19	200	16	1
Linguine, Dreamfields	1 cup	42	37	5	190	7	1
Penne, Atkins	1 cup	13	8	5	210	29	3
Penne, Dreamfields	1 cup	42	37	5	190		1
Penne, Mueller's	1 cup	31	12	19	200	16	1
Rotini, Atkins	1 cup	13	8	5	210	29	3
Rotini, Mueller's	1 cup	31	12	19	200	16	1
Spaghetti, Atkins	1 cup	13	8	5	210	29	3
Spaghetti, Carb Fit	1 cup	17	8	9	210	26	4
Spaghetti, Dreamfields	1 cup	42	37	5	190	7	1

PIZZA

When it comes to choosing between pizza and your low-carb way of eating, pizza often wins. That's not surprising—the average American eats more than 20 pounds of pizza every year. Nationwide, Americans eat enough pizza every day to cover 100 acres! And two of the top 10 fast-food restaurants are pizza chains (see the Fast Food section of this book for more information). Pizza is so popular and convenient that it's hard to avoid. What to do? Here's one idea: Save pizza as a treat for special occasions.

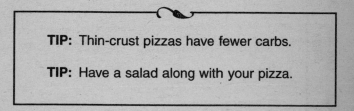

TIP: Thin-crust pizzas have fewer carbs.

TIP: Have a salad along with your pizza.

Food	Serving size	Carbohy-drates	Fiber	Net Carbs	Calories	Protein	Fat
Bacon cheeseburger, Tombstone	¼ pizza	39	8	31	408	18	20
BBQ chicken, Tombstone	½ pizza	38	9	29	320	15	12
Cheese, Jeno's	½ pizza	52	2	50	460	19	19
Cheese, Pizza for One, Celeste	1 pizza	42	6	36	390	13	19
Cheese, Totino's	½ pizza	39	2	37	370	17	16
Deluxe, Pizza for One, Celeste	1 pizza	42	6	36	431	14	23
Four cheese, Di Giorno	1 slice	39	3	36	320	16	11
Four cheese, Hot Pockets	1 pocket	41	3	38	392	12	20
French bread pizza, cheese, Healthy Choice	1 pizza	57	5	52	360	20	5
French bread pizza, pepperoni, Marie Callender's	1 pizza	50	4	46	570	29	28
Pepperoni, deep dish, Di Giorno	1 slice	32	3	29	395	17	22
Pepperoni, deep dish, Red Baron	½ pizza	48	0	48	480	16	25
Pepperoni, Hot Pockets	1 pocket	41	3	38	361	11	17
Pepperoni, Lean Pockets	1 pocket	42	3	39	287	14	7
Pepperoni, large, Tombstone	½ pizza	28	0	28	312	15	16
Pizza rolls, sausage, Totino's	6 rolls	24	1	23	230	8	11

Food	Serving size	Carbohy-drates	Fiber	Net Carbs	Calories	Protein	Fat
Sausage, deep dish, Jeno's	½ pizza	51	2	49	480	16	24
Sausage, Hot Pockets	1 pocket	37	3	34	363	11	19
Sausage, pepper, Pizza for One, Celeste	1 pizza	44	6	38	496	17	28
Sausage, pepperoni, Hot Pockets	1 pocket	38	3	35	376	11	20
Sausage, Pepperoni, Lean Pockets	1 pocket	41	4	38	279	13	7
Supreme, large, Di Giorno	1 slice	41	3	38	366	17	15
Supreme, Pizza for One, Celeste	1 pizza	44	6	38	500	18	28
Supreme, thin crispy crust, Di Giorno	1 slice	36	3	33	308	14	12
Zesty chicken supreme, Pizza for One, Celeste	1 pizza	40	6	34	360	14	16
REDUCED-CARB PRODUCTS							
French bread pizza, Carb Works, Red Baron	1 pizza	27	14	13	360	27	18
Pepperoni, Atkins	1 pizza	22	11	11	440	35	25
Pizza crust mix, Carb Fit	1 slice	7	2	5	100	20	3

Food	Serving size	Carbohy-drates	Fiber	Net Carbs	Calories	Protein	Fat
Pizza crust mix, MiniCarb	1 slice	6	3	3	130	18	5
Smokehouse, Atkins	1 pizza	22	11	11	420	34	23
Supreme, Atkins	1 pizza	22	11	11	360	30	19
Ultra Supreme, Lean Pockets	1 pocket	19	7	12	200	24	6

PORK

Juicy chops, crispy bacon, tender ham—pork is a favorite food for the low-carb lifestyle. Contrary to popular belief, you don't have to eat a lot of bacon if you're following a low-carb diet! (But you can eat more of it than low-fat diets allow.) Choose your favorite pork cuts and enjoy them without guilt.

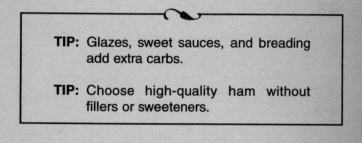

TIP: Glazes, sweet sauces, and breading add extra carbs.

TIP: Choose high-quality ham without fillers or sweeteners.

Food	Serving size	Carbohy-drates	Fiber	Net Carbs	Calories	Protein	Fat
(all portions are cooked)							
Arm, braised	3 oz.	0	0	0	280	24	20
Arm, roasted	3 oz.	0	0	0	269	20	20
Bacon, Canadian-style	2 slices	1	0	1	87	11	4
Bacon	3 strips	0	0	0	378	6	35
Chops, center loin, braised	3 oz.	0	0	0	210	24	12
Chops, center loin, broiled	3 oz.	0	0	0	204	24	11
Chops, center loin, pan fried	3 oz.	0	0	0	235	25	14
Chops, center rib, braised	3 oz.	0	0	0	213	23	13
Chops, center rib, broiled	3 oz.	0	0	0	224	25	13
Chops, center rib, pan fried	3 oz.	0	0	0	190	24	10
Chops, loin blade, braised	3 oz.	0	0	0	275	19	22
Chops, loin blade, broiled	3 oz.	0	0	0	272	19	21
Chops, loin blade, pan fried	3 oz.	0	0	0	291	19	24
Ham, cured, canned	3 oz.	0	0	0	102	16	4
Ham, cured, center slice	3 oz.	0	0	0	173	17	11
Ham, cured, roasted	3 oz.	0	0	0	151	19	8

Food	Serving size	Carbohy-drates	Fiber	Net Carbs	Calories	Protein	Fat
Ham steak, cured	3 oz.	0	0	0	104	17	4
Loin, braised	3 oz.	0	0	0	203	23	12
Loin, roasted	3 oz.	0	0	0	211	23	13
Picnic, braised	3 oz.	0	0	0	280	24	20
Roast, center loin, roasted	3 oz.	0	0	0	199	22	11
Roast, center rib, roasted	3 oz.	0	0	0	217	23	13
Sausage, fresh	3 oz.	0	0	0	100	5	8
Spareribs	3 oz.	0	0	0	337	25	26
Tenderloin, broiled	3 oz.	0	0	0	171	25	7
Tenderloin, roasted	3 oz.	0	0	0	147	24	5

POULTRY

Low-carb cookbooks are full of fast, simple, and delicious chicken recipes. A boneless chicken breast, for instance, can be turned into a low-carb stir-fry with plenty of vegetables in under half an hour. Baked drumsticks or wings are easy to prepare in advance and make a great snack or quick lunch. Watch out for fried chicken and chicken nuggets, however—even a small serving is high in added carbs. Turkey legs, wings, and breasts are now sold separately at the butcher counter, so even individuals and small families can enjoy home-cooked turkey without enduring days of leftovers.

TIP: For safe food handling, keep uncooked poultry away from foods that will be served raw.

TIP: The coating on fried chicken is high in carbs.

Food	Serving size	Carbohydrates	Fiber	Net Carbs	Calories	Protein	Fat
(all portions are cooked)							
Buffalo wings, frozen, Tyson's	1 piece	0	0	0	55	5	4
Chicken, boneless breast, fried, batter dipped	½ breast (3.5 oz.)	9	0	9	260	25	13
Chicken breast, fried	½ breast (3.5 oz.)	2	0	2	218	31	9
Chicken breast, roasted	½ breast (3.5 oz.)	0	0	0	193	29	8
Chicken breast, stewed	½ breast (3.5 oz.)	0	0	0	202	30	8
Chicken drumstick, fried	1 drumstick	1	0	1	120	13	7
Chicken drumstick, roasted	1 drumstick	0	0	0	112	14	6
Chicken drumstick, stewed	1 drumstick	0	0	0	116	14	6
Chicken leg, fried	1 leg (4 oz.)	3	0	3	284	30	16
Chicken leg, roasted	1 leg (4 oz.)	0	0	0	264	30	15
Chicken leg, stewed	1 leg (4 oz.)	0	0	0	275	30	15
Chicken liver, braised	3.5 oz.	1	0	1	157	24	6

Food	Serving size	Carbohydrates	Fiber	Net Carbs	Calories	Protein	Fat
Chicken nuggets, frozen, Banquet	5 pieces	13	1	12	276	11	20
Chicken nuggets, frozen, Perdue	5 pieces	12	0	12	177	12	9
Chicken nuggets, frozen, Tyson	5 pieces	20	0	20	280	15	15
Chicken thigh, fried	1 thigh (2.2 oz.)	2	0	2	162	17	9
Chicken thigh, roasted	1 thigh (2.2 oz.)	0	0	0	153	16	10
Chicken thigh, stewed	1 thigh (2.2 oz.)	0	0	0	158	16	10
Chicken wing, fried	1 wing (1 oz.)	1	0	1	103	8	7
Chicken wing, roasted	1 wing (1 oz.)	0	0	0	99	9	7
Chicken wing, stewed	1 wing (1 oz.)	0	0	0	100	9	7
Cornish game hen, roasted	3.5 oz.	0	0	0	231	19	16
Duck, roasted, no skin	3.5 oz.	0	0	0	201	24	11
Duck, roasted, skin	3.5 oz.	0	0	0	337	19	28
Turkey bacon	1 slice	0	0	0	34	2	3
Turkey, breast, no skin, roasted	3.5 oz.	0	0	0	157	30	3
Turkey, breast, skin, roasted	3.5 oz.	0	0	0	197	28	8
Turkey, dark meat, roasted, no skin	3.5 oz.	0	0	0	187	29	7
Turkey, dark meat, roasted, skin	3.5 oz.	0	0	0	221	28	12
Turkey, ground	3.5 oz.	0	0	0	170	21	10

PUDDING, CUSTARD, AND GELATIN

Favorite desserts such as pudding, custard, and Jell-O® can still easily be part of your low-carb lifestyle. These desserts are quick and easy to make. The versions made with sweeteners provide a satisfying sweet treat with very few net carbs. Top your dessert with real whipped cream, not a prepared topping that could add a lot of extra carbs.

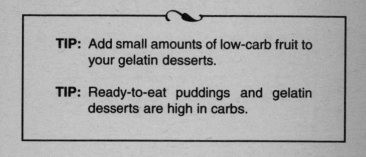

TIP: Add small amounts of low-carb fruit to your gelatin desserts.

TIP: Ready-to-eat puddings and gelatin desserts are high in carbs.

Food	Serving size	Carbohy-drates	Fiber	Net Carbs	Calories	Protein	Fat
Banana pudding, regular mix, whole milk	4 oz.	26	0	26	155	4	4
Bread pudding	4 oz.	40	0	40	250	5	8
Chocolate pudding, Kozy Shack	4 oz.	24	1	23	140	3	4
Chocolate pudding, Handi-Snacks	3.5 oz.	21	1	20	120	1	4
Chocolate pudding, Handi-Snacks, fat-free	3.5 oz.	21	0	21	92	2	0
Chocolate pudding, Jell-O	4 oz.	32	1	32	189	3	5
Chocolate pudding, regular mix, whole milk	4 oz.	26	1	25	158	5	5
Custard, egg, mix, whole milk	4 oz.	23	0	23	161	5	5
Flan/crème caramel, mix, whole milk	4 oz.	25	0	25	150	4	4
Jell-O, regular	0.7 oz.	19	0	19	84	2	0
Jell-O, fat-free	0.7 oz.	19	0	19	84	2	0
Jell-O, sugar-free	0.7 oz.	0	0	0	4	1	0
Jell-O Pudding Smoothie Snacks	4 oz.	18	0	18	99	1	3
Jell-O sugar-free pudding, chocolate	4 oz.	7	1	6	90	1	0
Jell-O sugar-free pudding, vanilla	4 oz.	5	0	5	80	0	0
Rice pudding, Kozy Shack	4 oz.	23	1	22	130	4	3
Rice pudding, regular mix, whole milk	4 oz.	30	0	30	174	5	4

Food	Serving size	Carbohy- drates	Fiber	Net Carbs	Calories	Protein	Fat
Tapioca pudding, Handi-Snacks	3.5 oz.	20	1	19	116	1	4
Tapioca pudding, Kozy Shack	4 oz.	25	0	25	140	3	3
Tapioca pudding, fat-free, Jell-O	4 oz.	23	0	23	96	1	0
Tapioca pudding, regular mix, whole milk	4 oz.	27	0	27	162	4	4
Vanilla pudding, Handi-Snacks	3.5 oz.	20	1	19	114	1	4
Vanilla pudding, Kozy Shack	4 oz.	22	0	22	130	3	3
Vanilla pudding, regular mix, whole milk	4 oz.	26	0	26	155	4	4

SALAD DRESSINGS

When you follow the low-carb approach, you start eating a *lot* more salad. That means more healthy vegetables in your diet—and more salad dressing. Traditional low-fat dieters are told avoid salad dressing or choose low-fat versions, but on a low-carb diet it's OK to enjoy creamy dressings. In fact, you have to watch out for the reduced-fat dressings. Many of these products replace the missing flavor with sweeteners that add carbs.

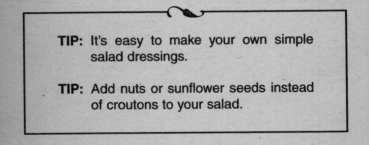

TIP: It's easy to make your own simple salad dressings.

TIP: Add nuts or sunflower seeds instead of croutons to your salad.

Food	Serving size	Carbohy-drates	Fiber	Net Carbs	Calories	Protein	Fat
Balsamic vinaigrette, Annie's	1 T	2	0	2	50	0	5
Balsamic vinegar, Newman's Own	1 T	2	0	2	44	0	4
Blue cheese	1 T	1	0	1	76	1	8
Blue cheese, chunky, Seven Seas	1 T	3	0	3	45	0	4
Blue cheese, chunky, Wish-Bone	1 T	1	0	1	85	0	8
Blue cheese, chunky, fat free, Wish-Bone	1 T	4	0	4	18	0	0
Caesar	1 T	1	0	2	60	1	6
Caesar, classic, Wish-Bone	1 T	1	0	1	55	0	5
Caesar, creamy, Newman's Own	1 T	1	0	1	84	0	9
Caesar, creamy, Wish-Bone	1 T	1	0	1	90	0	9
Caesar, Kraft	1 T	1	0	1	65	0	7
French	1 T	3	0	3	69	0	7
French, Annie's Naturals	1 T	2	0	2	45	0	5
French, creamy, Kraft	1 T	5	0	5	155	0	15
French, Kraft	1 T	2	0	2	60	0	6
French, Wish-Bone	1 T	3	0	3	60	0	6
French, low-fat	1 T	2	0	2	21	0	1

Food	Serving size	Carbohy-drates	Fiber	Net Carbs	Calories	Protein	Fat
Garlic, creamy, Kraft	1 T	2	0	2	55	0	6
Green goddess, Seven Seas	1 T	1	0	1	60	0	7
Honey dijon, fat free, Kraft	1 T	10	0	10	44	1	0
Honey dijon, fat free, Wish-Bone	1 T	5	0	5	28	1	0
Honey dijon, Kraft	1 T	6	0	6	114	0	10
Honey mustard, Annie's Naturals	1 T	3	0	3	23	0	1
Italian	1 T	2	0	2	69	0	7
Italian, creamy, Kraft	1 T	2	0	2	107	0	11
Italian, creamy, Wish-Bone	1 T	2	0	2	55	0	5
Italian, fat free, Kraft	1 T	2	0	2	10	0	0
Italian, fat free, Seven Seas	1 T	1	0	1	5	0	0
Italian, fat free, Wish-Bone	1 T	3	0	3	10	0	0
Italian, herb and cheese, Hidden Valley	1 T	3	0	3	15	1	0
Italian, low-fat	1 T	1	0	1	16	0	2
Italian, Wish-Bone	1 T	2	0	2	40	0	4
Italian, zesty, Kraft	1 T	1	0	1	55	0	6
Ranch, buttermilk, Kraft	1 T	2	1	1	152	0	16

Food	Serving size	Carbohy-drates	Fiber	Net Carbs	Calories	Protein	Fat
Ranch, creamy, Hidden Valley	1 T	0	0	0	55	1	6
Ranch, fat free, Kraft	1 T	6	0	6	24	0	0
Ranch, fat free, Wish-Bone	1 T	4	0	4	15	0	0
Ranch, Kraft	1 T	1	0	1	75	0	8
Ranch, light original, Hidden Valley	1 T	2	0	2	40	1	4
Ranch, Newman's Own	1 T	1	0	1	90	1	10
Ranch, original, Hidden Valley	1 T	0	0	0	70	2	7
Ranch, spicy, Hidden Valley	1 T	1	0	1	67	0	7
Ranch, Wish-Bone	1 T	1	0	1	80	0	8
Roquefort	1 T	1	0	1	76	1	8
Russian	1 T	2	0	2	74	0	8
Russian, Kraft	1 T	5	0	5	65	0	5
Russian, low fat	1 T	4	0	4	23	0	1
Russian, Wish-Bone	1 T	8	0	8	55	0	3
Thousand island	1 T	2	0	2	60	0	6
Thousand island, Annie's Naturals	1 T	3	0	3	45	0	4
Thousand island, fat free, Kraft	1 T	9	0	9	36	0	0

Food	Serving size	Carbohy-drates	Fiber	Net Carbs	Calories	Protein	Fat
Thousand island, fat free, Wish-Bone	1 T	5	0	5	18	0	0
Thousand island, Kraft	1 T	5	0	5	110	0	10
Thousand island, low fat	1 T	2	0	2	24	0	2
Thousand island, Wish-Bone	1 T	9	0	9	70	0	6
Vinaigrette, balsamic, Wish-Bone	1 T	2	0	2	30	0	3
Vinaigrette, red wine, fat free, Wish-Bone	1 T	4	0	4	18	0	0
Vinaigrette, red wine, Wish-Bone	1 T	5	0	5	45	0	3
Vinegar and oil	1 T	0	0	0	72	0	8
Viva Italian, Seven Seas	1 T	1	0	1	55	0	6

REDUCED-CARB PRODUCTS

Food	Serving size	Carbohy-drates	Fiber	Net Carbs	Calories	Protein	Fat
Blue cheese, Carb Options	1 T	0	0	0	75	0	8
Blue cheese, CarbWell	1 T	0	0	0	60	0	7
Caesar, classic, CarbWell	1 T	0	0	0	52	0	6
French, country, Atkins	1 T	0	0	0	50	0	6
Honey mustard, Atkins	1 T	0	0	0	55	0	6

Food	Serving size	Carbohy-drates	Fiber	Net Carbs	Calories	Protein	Fat
Italian, Carb Options	1 T	0	0	0	35	0	4
Italian, CarbWell	1 T	0	0	0	36	0	4
Lemon poppyseed, Atkins	1 T	0	0	0	50	0	6
Ranch, Carb Options	1 T	0	0	0	75	0	9

SHAKES AND NUTRITIONAL DRINKS

When you're on the go and can't stop for a real meal, shake mixes or ready-to-drink shakes are a good alternative to grabbing a fast-food meal; they're also a great between-meals snack. These drinks generally have high amounts of protein, vitamins, and minerals, and they're low in fat, but they can be on the high side for net carbs. If you need to really watch your net carbs, choose one of the reduced-carb products.

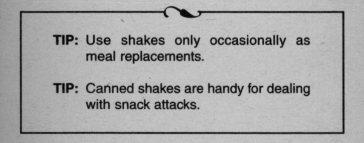

TIP: Use shakes only occasionally as meal replacements.

TIP: Canned shakes are handy for dealing with snack attacks.

Food	Serving size	Carbohy-drates	Fiber	Net Carbs	Calories	Protein	Fat
Carnation Instant Breakfast, cappuccino	1 packet	26	0	26	124	5	0
Carnation Instant Breakfast, chocolate malt	1 packet	27	1	26	133	4	1
Carnation Instant Breakfast, milk chocolate	1 packet	27	1	26	137	5	1
Ensure, all flavors	8 fl. oz.	50	0	50	351	13	11
GoLean, chocolate	1 can (11 fl. oz.)	38	7	31	239	15	3
GoLean, vanilla	1 can (11 fl. oz.)	36	7	29	227	15	3
Met-Rx, vanilla	1 can (11 fl. oz.)	19	1	18	203	25	3
Slim-Fast, French vanilla	1 can (11 fl. oz.)	40	5	35	223	10	3
Slim-Fast, milk chocolate	1 can (11 fl. oz.)	40	5	35	227	10	3
Ultra Slim-Fast, chocolate malt mix	1 serving (2 scoops)	24	5	19	120	5	1
Ultra Slim-Fast, chocolate royale mix	1 serving (2 scoops)	24	5	19	120	5	1

Food	Serving size	Carbohy-drates	Fiber	Net Carbs	Calories	Protein	Fat
Ultra Slim-Fast, French vanilla mix	1 serving (2 scoops)	25	5	20	120	5	1
Ultra Slim-Fast, milk chocolate mix	1 serving (2 scoops)	23	5	18	120	20	1
Ultra Slim-Fast, strawberry mix	1 serving (2 scoops)	25	4	21	120	5	1
Zone Perfect, Dutch chocolate	1 can (8 fl. oz.)	31	4	27	281	19	9
Zone Perfect, French vanilla	1 can (8 fl. oz.)	29	4	25	260	18	8
REDUCED-CARB PRODUCTS							
Atkins, café au lait	1 can (11 fl. oz.)	5	3	2	170	20	9
Atkins, cappuccino mix	1 serving (2 scoops)	10	7	3	140	15	4
Atkins, chocolate mix	1 serving (2 scoops)	10	7	3	140	15	4
Atkins, chocolate delight	1 can (11 fl. oz.)	4	3	1	170	20	9
Atkins, chocolate royale	1 can (11 fl. oz.)	6	4	2	170	20	9

Food	Serving size	Carbohy-drates	Fiber	Net Carbs	Calories	Protein	Fat
Atkins, strawberry	1 can (11 fl. oz.)	4	2	2	170	20	9
Atkins, strawberry mix	1 serving (2 scoops)	9	6	3	130	15	4
Atkins, vanilla	1 can (11 fl. oz.)	4	3	1	170	20	9
Atkins, vanilla mix	1 serving (2 scoops)	9	6	3	130	15	4
Carb Options, chocolate	1 can (11 fl. oz.)	6	4	2	190	20	9
Carb Options, vanilla	1 can (11 fl. oz.)	6	4	2	190	20	9
Carb Solutions, chocolate	1 can (11 fl. oz.)	5	3	2	110	21	1
Carborite, banana mix	1 serving (2 scoops)	5	3	2	135	24	3
Carborite, chocolate mix	1 serving (2 scoops)	5	3	2	135	24	3
Carborite, strawberry mix	1 serving (2 scoops)	5	3	2	135	24	3
Carborite, vanilla mix	1 serving (2 scoops)	5	3	2	135	24	3

Food	Serving size	Carbohy-drates	Fiber	Net Carbs	Calories	Protein	Fat
Carb Solutions, chocolate mix	1 serving (2 scoops)	5	2	3	123	20	3
Carb Solutions, vanilla	1 can (11 fl. oz.)	4	2	2	100	21	1
Carb Solutions, vanilla mix	1 serving (2 scoops)	3	0	3	119	21	3

SNACK FOODS

Salty snack foods are the downfall of many a dieter. In addition to the large amounts of low-quality carbs in these foods, they're very high in salt and fat and may contain dangerous trans fats. But even when you know they're not the best choice, these crispy snacks are very difficult to resist. Today's low-carb alternatives make resisting easier by giving you better choices, with more crunch and flavor but with fewer carbs.

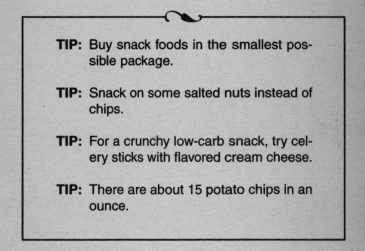

TIP: Buy snack foods in the smallest possible package.

TIP: Snack on some salted nuts instead of chips.

TIP: For a crunchy low-carb snack, try celery sticks with flavored cream cheese.

TIP: There are about 15 potato chips in an ounce.

Food	Serving size	Carbohy-drates	Fiber	Net Carbs	Calories	Protein	Fat
Beef jerky	1 large piece	2	0	2	82	7	5
Bugles	1 oz.	18	0	18	156	1	9
Bugles, baked	1 oz.	27	0	27	150	2	4
Cheese puffs	1 oz.	15	0	15	157	2	10
Cheetos	1 oz.	15	0	15	159	2	10
Chex Mix	1 oz.	19	2	17	120	3	5
Combos	1 oz.	20	0	20	139	3	5
Corn chip	1 oz.	16	1	15	153	2	10
Fritos corn chips	1 oz.	15	1	14	158	2	10
Popcorn cake	1 cake	8	0	8	38	1	0
Popcorn, caramel	1 oz.	22	2	20	122	1	4
Popcorn, caramel, peanuts	1 oz.	23	1	22	113	2	2
Popcorn, cheese	1 oz.	15	3	12	149	3	9
Popcorn, plain, air-popped	1 oz.	22	4	18	108	3	1
Popcorn, plain, oil-popped	1 oz.	16	3	13	142	3	8
Pork rinds	1 oz.	2	0	2	157	15	10
Potato chips	1 oz.	15	1	14	152	2	10

Food	Serving size	Carbohy-drates	Fiber	Net Carbs	Calories	Protein	Fat
Potato chips, barbeque	1 oz.	15	1	14	139	2	9
Potato chips, light	1 oz.	19	2	17	134	2	6
Potato chips, sour cream and onion	1 oz.	15	2	13	151	2	10
Pretzels	2 oz.	48	2	46	229	6	2
Rice cakes	1 cake	7	0	7	35	1	0
Soy Crisps, GeniSoy	1 oz.	18	2	16	120	6	3
Sunchips, multigrain	1 oz.	19	2	17	137	2	6
Taro chips	1 oz.	16	2	15	115	1	6
Tortilla chips	1 oz.	18	2	16	142	2	7
Tortilla chips, nacho	1 oz.	18	2	16	141	2	7

REDUCED-CARB PRODUCTS

Food	Serving size	Carbohy-drates	Fiber	Net Carbs	Calories	Protein	Fat
Bar-B-Que chips, Carb Solutions	1 oz.	4	0	4	130	19	5
BBQ Snack Chips, Carb Options	1 oz.	9	4	5	100	12	4
Cheese puffs, Carb Fit	1 oz.	7	1	6	140	10	8
Crunchers, BBQ, Atkins	1 oz.	8	4	4	100	13	3
Crunchers, sour cream and onions, Atkins	1 oz.	8	3	5	100	12	4

Food	Serving size	Carbohy-drates	Fiber	Net Carbs	Calories	Protein	Fat
Nacho Cheese chips, Carb Solutions	1 oz.	3	0	3	130	19	5
Nacho chips, Carb Options	1 oz.	8	4	4	110	12	5
Pretzels, Carb Fit	1 oz.	10	3	7	120	10	4
Ranch Snack chips, Carb Options	1 oz.	8	4	4	110	12	5
Soy nuts, Carb Fit	½ cup	11	5	6	140	11	6
Soy pretzels, CarbSense	1 oz.	12	4	8	100	10	3
Soy thins, MiniCarb	1 oz.	8	3	5	120	12	5
Soy tortilla chips, CarbSense	1 oz.	12	4	8	140	5	8
Tortilla chips, Carb Fit	1 oz.	9	4	5	150	9	8

SOUP

Soup is the dieter's best friend. A cup of hot vegetable soup, for instance, makes a satisfying low-carb snack that also sneaks in some of your daily vegetable quota. Hot soup puts a temporary hold on hunger pangs, so you can resist other between-meal snacks. And a cup of low-carb soup before the main course at a meal fills you up and helps you stay away from high-carb temptations.

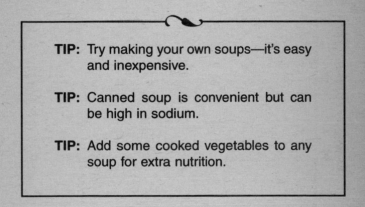

TIP: Try making your own soups—it's easy and inexpensive.

TIP: Canned soup is convenient but can be high in sodium.

TIP: Add some cooked vegetables to any soup for extra nutrition.

Food	Serving size	Carbohy-drates	Fiber	Net Carbs	Calories	Protein	Fat
(all soups are prepared)							
Asparagus, cream of	8 fl. oz.	11	0	11	85	2	4
Bean with ham, chunky	8 fl. oz.	27	11	16	231	13	9
Beef barley, Progresso	8 fl. oz.	13	3	10	130	10	4
Beef broth	8 fl. oz.	2	0	2	29	5	0
Beef noodle	8 fl. oz.	9	0	9	83	5	3
Beef vegetable, Progresso	8 fl. oz.	13	2	11	120	10	3
Black bean	8 fl. oz.	20	4	16	116	6	2
Black bean with rice, Pritikin	8 fl. oz.	37	0	37	200	11	1
Broccoli and cheese, Lipton Cup-A-Soup	1 serving	9	1	8	67	2	3
Celery, cream of	8 fl. oz.	16	1	15	161	6	8
Cheese	8 fl. oz.	11	1	10	156	5	10
Chickarina, Progresso	8 fl. oz.	12	0	12	130	8	5
Chicken broth	8 fl. oz.	1	0	1	38	5	1
Chicken, cream of	8 fl. oz.	9	0	9	117	3	7
Chicken, cream of, Lipton Cup-A-Soup	1 serving	12	1	11	68	1	2
Chicken gumbo	8 fl. oz.	8	2	6	56	3	1

Food	Serving size	Carbohy-drates	Fiber	Net Carbs	Calories	Protein	Fat
Chicken mushroom	8 fl. oz.	9	0	9	132	4	9
Chicken noodle	8 fl. oz.	9	1	8	75	4	3
Chicken noodle, Lipton Cup-A-Soup	1 serving	10	0	10	61	3	1
Chicken noodle, Progresso	8 fl. oz.	12	1	11	110	10	2
Chicken pasta, Pritikin	8 fl. oz.	15	0	15	80	5	0
Chicken pasta, fat free, Lipton Cup-A-Soup	1 serving	8	0	8	44	2	0
Chicken rice	8 fl. oz.	7	1	6	60	4	2
Chicken rice with vegetables, Progresso	8 fl. oz.	13	1	12	90	6	2
Chicken vegetable	8 fl. oz.	9	1	8	75	4	3
Chicken vegetable, Lipton Cup-A-Soup	1 serving	10	0	10	52	1	1
Clam chowder, Manhattan	8 fl. oz.	12	2	10	78	2	2
Clam chowder, New England	8 fl. oz.	12	2	10	95	5	3
Creamy broccoli, Slim-Fast	1 container	30	5	25	205	10	5
Creamy potato cheddar, Slim-Fast	1 container	35	5	30	225	10	5
Creamy tomato, Progresso	8 fl. oz.	30	1	29	190	4	6
Gazpacho	8 fl. oz.	4	1	3	46	7	0

Food	Serving size	Carbohy-drates	Fiber	Net Carbs	Calories	Protein	Fat
Lentil, Progresso	8 fl. oz.	22	7	15	140	9	2
Minestrone	8 fl. oz.	11	1	10	82	4	3
Minestrone, Pritikin	8 fl. oz.	18	0	18	89	3	0
Minestrone, Progresso	8 fl. oz.	21	5	16	120	5	2
Mushroom barley	8 fl. oz.	12	1	11	73	2	2
Mushroom, cream of	8 fl. oz.	9	1	8	129	2	9
Onion	8 fl. oz.	8	1	7	58	4	2
Onion, cream of	8 fl. oz.	13	1	12	107	3	5
Oyster stew	8 fl. oz.	4	0	4	58	2	4
Pea, green	8 fl. oz.	26	3	23	165	9	3
Pea, split, Pritikin	8 fl. oz.	32	0	32	181	12	0
Pea, split with ham	8 fl. oz.	28	2	26	190	10	4
Pea, split with ham, Progresso	8 fl. oz.	20	5	15	150	9	4
Pepperpot	8 fl. oz.	9	1	8	104	6	5
Potato, cream of	8 fl. oz.	12	0	12	73	2	2
Ramen noodles, beef, Maruchan	1 serving	26	0	26	190	5	8
Ramen noodles, chicken, Maruchan	1 serving	26	0	26	190	5	8

Food	Serving size	Carbohy-drates	Fiber	Net Carbs	Calories	Protein	Fat
Ramen noodles, chicken, Nissin Cup	1 container	37	0	37	296	6	14
Ramen noodles, oriental, Oodles of Noodles	1 serving	28	0	28	190	4	7
Ramen noodles, pork, Maruchan	1 serving	26	0	26	180	5	8
Ramen noodles, shrimp, Maruchan	1.5 oz.	26	0	26	190	5	8
Shrimp, cream of	8 fl. oz.	8	0	8	90	3	5
Tomato	8 fl. oz.	17	1	16	85	2	2
Tomato, Lipton Cup-A-Soup	1 serving	20	1	19	95	2	1
Tomato bisque	8 fl. oz.	24	1	23	124	2	3
Tomato rice	8 fl. oz.	22	2	20	119	2	3
Turkey noodle	8 fl. oz.	9	1	8	68	4	2
Turkey vegetable	8 fl. oz.	9	1	8	72	3	3
Vegetable, Pritikin	8 fl. oz.	16	0	16	89	5	0
Vegetable beef	8 fl. oz.	10	1	9	78	6	2
Vegetable, spring, Lipton Cup-A-Soup	1 serving	8	0	8	45	2	1
Vegetarian vegetable	8 fl. oz.	12	1	11	72	2	2

REDUCED-CARB PRODUCTS

Food	Serving size	Carbohy-drates	Fiber	Net Carbs	Calories	Protein	Fat
Bacon, cheese, Atkins	½ cup	9	5	4	120	12	4
Beef vegetable, Progresso Carb Monitor	8 fl. oz.	6	1	5	70	8	2
Broccoli cheese, Atkins	8 fl. oz.	3	2	1	78	5	5
Chicken broccoli cheese, Campbell's Carb Request	8 fl. oz.	8	5	3	130	9	7
Chicken cheese enchilada, Atkins	8 fl. oz.	4	2	2	94	5	6
Chicken cheese enchilada style, Progresso Carb Monitor	8 fl. oz.	7	1	6	208	9	16
Chicken noodle, Atkins	8 fl. oz.	3	1	2	40	4	1
Chicken vegetable, Progresso Carb Monitor	8 fl. oz.	7	1	6	74	7	2
Cream of mushroom, Atkins	8 fl. oz.	2	0	2	51	2	4
Mediterranean meatball, Campbell's Carb Request	8 fl. oz.	5	2	3	90	8	5
Roasted chicken, penne, Campbell's Carb Request	8 fl. oz.	7	2	5	70	9	1

Food	Serving size	Carbohy-drates	Fiber	Net Carbs	Calories	Protein	Fat
Savory beef, mushroom, Campbell's Carb Request	8 fl. oz.	7	1	6	70	7	2
Spicy sausage, chicken, Campbell's Carb Request	8 fl. oz.	7	2	5	100	8	4
Vegetable, Atkins	½ cup	9	5	4	90	11	1

SOY FOODS

Because soy is high in vegetable protein, very low in fat, and has few net carbs, it's a great food for health-conscious people. Soy products are also very useful for vegetarians and others who want to follow a low-carb diet but don't want to eat meat or other animal foods. But like any other food, processed soy products can have more carbs than you realize. Plain soy milk is slightly lower in carbs than cow's milk, for example, but flavored soy milk has a lot more carbs! Read the labels and be aware of portion size.

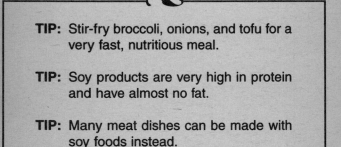

TIP: Stir-fry broccoli, onions, and tofu for a very fast, nutritious meal.

TIP: Soy products are very high in protein and have almost no fat.

TIP: Many meat dishes can be made with soy foods instead.

Food	Serving size	Carbohy-drates	Fiber	Net Carbs	Calories	Protein	Fat
Breakfast Links, Boca	2 links	5	2	3	90	10	3
Breakfast Links, Morningstar Farms	1 link	3	2	1	78	9	3
Burger, All-American, Boca	1 patty	5	4	1	90	13	4
Burger, Better 'n Burgers, Morningstar Farms	1 patty	8	4	4	91	14	1
Burger, grilled vegetable, Boca	1 patty	6	5	1	80	13	1
Burger, Grillers, Morningstar Farms	1 patty	4	2	2	160	17	8
Burger, Harvest Burger, Green Giant	1 patty	7	6	1	138	18	4
Burger, spicy black bean, Morningstar Farms	1 patty	15	5	10	115	12	1
Burger, vegan, Natural Touch	1 patty	8	4	4	91	14	1
Chai beverage, WestSoy	8 fl. oz.	25	0	25	130	2	3
Chicken nuggets, Morningstar Farms	3 oz.	18	4	14	184	13	7
Chicken nuggets, Loma Linda	3 oz.	13	11	2	255	14	17
Chicken patty, Boca	1 patty	12	2	10	150	13	6
Chicken Supreme, Loma Linda	0.9 oz.	6	4	2	89	15	0
Chili, vegetarian, Natural Touch	8 oz.	26	13	13	176	16	1

Food	Serving size	Carbohy-drates	Fiber	Net Carbs	Calories	Protein	Fat
Corn dog, Loma Linda	1 corn dog	23	1	22	162	8	4
Corn dog, Morningstar Farms	1 corn dog	23	1	22	162	8	4
Country Stew, Worthington	8.5 oz.	18	4	15	205	13	9
Creamer, soy, Silk	1 T	1	0	1	15	0	1
Creamer, soy, French vanilla, Silk	1 T	3	0	3	20	0	0
Creamer, soy, hazelnut, Silk	1 T	1	0	1	15	0	0
Cutlets, Worthington	2.2 oz.	3	2	1	68	13	1
Deli Franks, Morningstar Farms	1 frank	4	3	1	112	10	6
Grillers, Morningstar Farms	1 patty	5	2	3	170	16	9
Ice cream, Better Pecan, Tofutti	4 oz.	22	0	22	210	1	13
Ice cream, Chocolate Supreme, Tofutti	4 oz.	18	0	18	180	3	11
Ice cream, mint chocolate chip, Tofutti	4 oz.	21	0	21	210	3	13
Ice cream, vanilla, Tofutti	4 oz.	20	0	20	190	2	11
Ice cream, Wildberry Supreme	4 oz.	24	0	24	190	2	9
Lasagna, Boca	10 oz.	41	4	36	270	20	5
Leanies, Worthington	1.4 oz.	3	2	1	100	8	7
Meatballs, Morningstar Farms	3 oz.	9	2	7	233	23	12

Food	Serving size	Carbohy-drates	Fiber	Net Carbs	Calories	Protein	Fat
Miso	1 cup	77	15	62	567	33	17
Multigrain Cutlets, Worthington	2.5 oz.	4	3	1	73	12	1
Natto	1 cup	25	10	15	371	31	19
Nine Bean Loaf, Natural Touch	3.2 oz.	15	4	11	154	8	7
Pizza, veggie supreme, Morningstar Farms	4.6 oz.	39	4	35	283	13	8
Salami, meatless, Worthington	2 oz.	3	2	1	121	13	7
Sausage, smoked, Boca	1 sausage	7	2	5	130	12	5
Savory Dinner Loaf, Loma Linda	0.9 oz.	7	5	2	91	14	1
Shake, chocolate, WestSoy	8 fl. oz.	30	4	26	170	7	4
Shake, Chocolate Delite with Soy, Ultra Slim-Fast	1 serving	25	5	20	170	15	2
Shake, soy chocolate, Slim-Fast	1 can	39	3	34	231	12	3
Shake, soy vanilla, Slim-Fast	1 can	38	5	33	227	12	3
Shake, vanilla, WestSoy	8 fl. oz.	28	3	25	170	7	3
Smoothie, banana berry, WestSoy	8 fl. oz.	28	2	26	140	3	2
Smoothie, Tropical Whip, WestSoy	8 fl. oz.	28	2	26	140	3	2

Food	Serving size	Carbohydrates	Fiber	Net Carbs	Calories	Protein	Fat
Soy cheese, American, Tofutti	1 slice	2	0	2	70	2	5
Soy cheese, mozzarella, Tofutti	1 slice	2	0	2	70	2	5
Soy cheese, roasted garlic, Tofutti	1 slice	2	0	2	70	2	5
Soy cream cheese, French onion, Tofutti	2 T	1	0	1	80	1	8
Soy cream cheese, garden veggie, Tofutti	2 T	1	0	1	80	1	8
Soy cream cheese, garlic herb, Tofutti	2 T	1	0	1	80	1	8
Soy cream cheese, herb chives, Tofutti	2 T	1	0	1	80	1	8
Soy cream cheese, plain, Tofutti	2 T	1	0	1	80	1	8
Soy cream cheese, salmon, Tofutti	2 T	1	0	1	80	1	8
Soy milk	8 fl. oz.	4	3	1	81	7	5
Soy milk, 8th Continent	8 fl oz.	8	0	8	80	7	3
Soy milk, WestSoy	8 fl. oz.	18	3	15	130	8	4
Soy milk, carob, Eden Soy	8 fl. oz.	27	0	27	170	7	4
Soy milk, chai, Silk	8 fl. oz.	20	1	19	130	7	3
Soy milk, chocolate, 8th Continent	8 fl. oz.	23	1	22	140	7	3
Soy milk, chocolate, Silk	8 fl. oz.	23	0	23	140	5	4
Soy milk, light, 8th Continent	8 fl. oz.	2	0	2	50	7	2

Food	Serving size	Carbohydrates	Fiber	Net Carbs	Calories	Protein	Fat
Soy milk, light, chocolate, 8ᵗʰ Continent	8 fl. oz.	13	0	13	90	7	2
Soy milk, mocha, Silk	8 fl. oz.	29	0	29	170	5	4
Soy milk, unsweetened, WestSoy	8 fl. oz.	5	4	1	90	9	5
Soy milk, unsweetened, chocolate, WestSoy	8 fl. oz.	6	5	1	100	9	5
Soy milk, unsweetened, vanilla, WestSoy	8 fl. oz.	5	4	1	100	9	5
Soy milk, vanilla, Edensoy	8 fl. oz.	24	1	23	150	7	3
Soy milk, vanilla, 8ᵗʰ Continent	8 fl. oz.	11	0	11	90	7	3
Soy milk, vanilla, light, 8ᵗʰ Continent	8 fl. oz.	5	0	5	60	7	1
Soy sour cream, Tofutti	2 T	9	0	9	85	1	7
Soy yogurt, blueberry, Silk	6 oz.	29	1	28	160	4	2
Soy yogurt, blueberry, Stonyfield Farm	6 oz.	33	4	29	170	7	2
Soy yogurt, chocolate, Stonyfield Farm	6 oz.	28	4	24	160	7	3
Soy yogurt, lemon, Silk	6 oz.	31	1	30	160	4	2
Soy yogurt, peach, Stonyfield Farm	6 oz.	32	4	28	170	7	2
Soy yogurt, plain, Silk	8 oz.	22	1	21	120	5	3
Soy yogurt, raspberry, Stonyfield Farm	6 oz.	32	4	28	170	7	2

Food	Serving size	Carbohy-drates	Fiber	Net Carbs	Calories	Protein	Fat
Soy yogurt, strawberry, Silk	6 oz.	31	1	30	160	4	2
Soy yogurt, strawberry, Stonyfield Farm	6 oz.	32	4	28	170	7	2
Soy yogurt, vanilla, Silk	6 oz.	23	1	22	120	4	2
Soy yogurt, vanilla, Stonyfield Farm	6 oz.	26	4	22	150	7	2
Tempeh	1 cup	16	0	16	320	31	18
Tofu, extra-firm	3 oz.	2	0	2	46	6	2
Tofu, firm	3 oz.	2	0	2	52	6	2
Tofu, soft	3 oz.	2	0	2	46	4	2
Turkee Slices, Worthington	3.3 oz.	5	0	5	193	13	14
Veggie Dog, Morningstar Farms	1 veggie dog	6	1	5	77	11	1

VEGETABLES

When you start eating the low-carb way, you start eating a lot of vegetables. That's because you're replacing low-quality carbs such as french fries with nutritious, delicious, low-carb vegetables such as sweet potatoes, broccoli, and salad greens. It's a change that's easy to make, because there's such an amazing variety of interesting vegetables to try.

TIP: The more colorful a vegetable is, the more nutrients it usually has.

TIP: Frozen vegetables are handy and just as nutritious as fresh.

TIP: Starchy vegetables such as corn are high in net carbs.

TIP: Sauces and glazes can add extra carbs to vegetable dishes.

TIP: Oven roasting brings out the flavor of root vegetables such as carrots.

TIP: Toss some extra veggies into soups, stews, and casseroles.

TIP: For a crunchy snack, try baby carrots, celery sticks, and other veggies.

Food	Serving size	Carbohy-drates	Fiber	Net Carbs	Calories	Protein	Fat
(all portions are cooked unless noted otherwise)							
Acorn squash, baked	1 cup	30	9	21	115	2	0
Acorn squash, mashed	1 cup	22	6	16	83	2	0
Alfalfa sprouts, raw	1 cup	1	1	0	10	1	0
Artichoke	1 medium	13	7	6	60	4	0
Arugala, raw	½ cup	0	0	0	3	0	0
Asian vegetables, sesame ginger sauce, Birds Eye	1 cup	12	2	10	60	2	1
Asparagus	½ cup	4	1	3	22	2	0
Asparagus, canned	1 cup	6	4	2	46	5	2
Asparagus stir-fry, Birds Eye	1 cup	15	2	13	80	3	0
Baby Brussels sprouts, butter sauce, Green Giant	1 cup	9	5	4	75	5	2
Baby corn, bean, pea mix, Birds Eye	¾ cup	13	2	11	79	2	0
Baby corn, vegetable blend, Birds Eye	⅔ cup	9	3	6	50	2	1
Baby lima beans, butter sauce, Green Giant	1 cup	30	6	24	165	8	2

Food	Serving size	Carbohy-drates	Fiber	Net Carbs	Calories	Protein	Fat
Baby mixed beans, carrots, Birds Eye	1 cup	6	2	4	35	1	0
Baby peas, vegetable blend, Birds Eye	¾ cup	7	2	5	40	2	0
Baby potato, vegetable blend, Birds Eye	¾ cup	8	1	7	40	1	0
Baby sweet peas, pearl onions	⅔ cup	12	3	9	60	4	0
Bamboo shoots, canned	1 cup	4	2	2	25	2	0
Beets, Harvard, canned, Green Giant	1 cup	45	6	39	180	0	0
Beets, sliced, canned	1 cup	16	4	12	70	2	0
Beets, sliced, pickled	1 cup	37	6	31	148	2	0
Broccoli, beans, onions, peppers, Birds Eye	1 cup	5	2	3	30	1	0
Broccoli, carrots, water chestnuts, Birds Eye	1 cup	6	2	4	35	1	0
Broccoli, cheese sauce, Birds Eye	½ cup	8	1	7	90	3	5
Broccoli, chopped	1 cup	10	6	4	52	6	0
Broccoli, raw, chopped	1 cup	5	3	2	25	3	0
Broccoli, rice, cheese sauce, Birds Eye	10 oz.	49	1	48	300	6	9
Broccoli, spears	½ cup	5	3	2	25	3	0

Food	Serving size	Carbohy-drates	Fiber	Net Carbs	Calories	Protein	Fat
Broccoli spears, butter sauce, Green Giant	1 cup	9	3	6	65	3	2
Brussels sprouts	1 cup	13	6	7	65	6	1
Burdock root	1 cup	26	2	24	110	3	0
Butternut squash, baked	1 cup	22	6	16	82	2	0
Butternut squash, mashed	1 cup	24	7	17	94	3	0
Cabbage, green, raw, shredded	1 cup	4	2	2	18	1	0
Cabbage, green, shredded	1 cup	7	4	3	34	2	0
Cabbage, red, raw, shredded	1 cup	4	1	3	19	1	0
Cabbage, red, shredded	1 cup	7	3	4	32	1	0
Cabbage, savoy, raw, shredded	1 cup	4	2	2	19	1	0
Cabbage, savoy, shredded	1 cup	8	4	4	35	3	0
California blend, cheddar sauce, Birds Eye	9.5 oz.	8	1	7	80	2	4
Carrots, baby, raw	1 medium	1	0	1	4	0	0
Carrots, honey glazed, Green Giant	1 cup	13	2	11	90	0	4
Carrots, raw	1 large	7	2	5	31	1	0
Carrots, sliced	1 cup	16	6	10	70	2	0

Food	Serving size	Carbohy-drates	Fiber	Net Carbs	Calories	Protein	Fat
Carrots, sliced, canned	1 cup	12	4	8	50	0	0
Cauliflower	½ cup	3	2	1	14	1	0
Cauliflower, carrots, snow pea pods, Birds Eye	1 cup	6	2	4	30	1	0
Cauliflower, cheese sauce, Green Giant	½ cup	7	1	6	60	2	3
Cauliflower, frozen	1 cup	7	5	2	34	3	0
Cauliflower, garlic sauce, Birds Eye	1 cup	5	2	3	55	2	4
Cauliflower, raw	1 cup	5	3	2	25	2	0
Celeriac (celery roots)	1 cup	9	2	7	42	2	0
Celery, raw	1 medium stalk	2	1	1	6	0	0
Chard, Swiss, chopped	1 cup	7	4	3	35	3	0
Chayote	1 cup	8	5	3	38	1	1
Chicory greens, raw, chopped	1 cup	9	7	2	41	3	0
Classic vegetable mix, Birds Eye	¾ cup	12	2	10	60	2	0
Collards, chopped	1 cup	9	5	4	49	4	1
Corn	1 ear	19	2	17	83	3	1
Corn, butter sauce, Birds Eye	½ cup	28	2	26	150	3	3

Food	Serving size	Carbohy-drates	Fiber	Net Carbs	Calories	Protein	Fat
Corn, cream style, canned, Green Giant	1 cup	44	2	42	200	4	1
Corn, kernels	1 cup	41	5	36	177	5	2
Corn, Niblets, butter sauce, Green Giant	1 cup	33	3	30	165	5	2
Corn, shoepeg, butter sauce, Green Giant	1 cup	28	4	24	147	4	3
Creamed corn, canned, Green Giant	1 cup	44	2	42	200	4	1
Creamed spinach, Birds Eye	½ cup	7	1	6	100	3	7
Cucumber, raw	1 medium	8	2	6	39	2	0
Dandelion greens, chopped	1 cup	7	3	4	35	2	0
Dandelion greens, chopped, raw	1 cup	5	2	3	27	2	0
Eggplant	1 cup	7	3	4	28	1	0
Endive, raw, chopped	½ cup	1	1	0	4	0	0
Fennel bulb, raw	1 cup	6	3	3	27	1	0
French fries	10 fries	16	2	14	100	2	4
French fries, golden crinkles, Ore-Ida	10 fries	18	2	16	152	2	8
Garden bean medley, toasted almonds, Birds Eye	1 cup	10	5	5	100	3	5
Garden medley, canned, Green Giant	1 cup	18	4	14	80	2	0

Food	Serving size	Carbohy-drates	Fiber	Net Carbs	Calories	Protein	Fat
Garlic, raw	3 cloves	3	0	3	13	1	0
Green beans	1 cup	10	4	6	44	2	0
Green bean stir-fry, Birds Eye	1 cup	19	2	17	100	4	0
Green beans, spaetzle, Birds Eye	1 cup	16	3	13	150	5	7
Hearts of palm, canned	1 cup	7	4	3	41	4	1
Hubbard squash, baked	1 cup	22	12	10	103	5	1
Hubbard squash, mashed	1 cup	15	7	8	71	4	1
Jerusalem artichoke, raw, sliced	1 cup	26	2	22	114	3	0
Jicama, raw, sliced	1 cup	11	6	5	46	1	0
Kale, chopped	1 cup	6	3	4	39	4	1
Kohlrabi	1 cup	11	2	9	48	3	0
Leeks, raw	1 cup	13	2	11	54	2	0
Lettuce, butterhead, raw, chopped	1 cup	1	1	0	7	1	0
Lettuce, iceberg, raw, chopped	1 cup	1	1	0	6	0	0
Lettuce, looseleaf, raw, shredded	½ cup	1	0	1	5	0	0
Lettuce, romaine, raw, shredded	½ cup	1	1	0	4	0	0
Mexicorn, Green Giant	1 cup	42	6	36	180	6	0

Food	Serving size	Carbohy-drates	Fiber	Net Carbs	Calories	Protein	Fat
Mung bean sprouts	1 cup	5	1	4	26	3	0
Mung bean sprouts, raw	1 cup	6	2	4	31	3	0
Mushrooms, crimini, raw	1 piece	1	0	1	3	0	0
Mushrooms, enoki, raw	1 large	0	0	0	2	0	0
Mushrooms, oyster	1 large	9	4	5	55	6	0
Mushrooms, portabella	1 medium	6	2	4	29	3	0
Mushrooms, shiitake	4 medium	10	2	8	40	1	0
Mushrooms, shiitake, dried	4 medium	11	2	9	44	1	0
Mushrooms, straw, canned	1 cup	9	5	4	58	7	1
Mushrooms, white, pieces	1 cup	8	3	5	42	3	1
Mushrooms, white, pieces, raw	½ cup	3	1	2	18	2	0
Mustard greens, chopped	1 cup	5	4	1	29	3	0
Okra, boiled	8 pods	6	2	4	27	2	0
Okra, sliced	½ cup	5	3	2	26	2	0
Onion, chopped	1 cup	21	3	18	92	3	0
Onion, chopped, raw	1 cup	14	3	11	61	2	0
Onion, green, raw	½ cup	4	2	2	16	1	0
Onion rings	10 rings	23	1	22	244	3	160

Food	Serving size	Carbohy-drates	Fiber	Net Carbs	Calories	Protein	Fat
Parsnip	1 parsnip	31	6	25	130	2	0
Pasta, vegetables, cheese sauce, Birds Eye	1 cup	27	1	26	170	7	4
Peas, pearl onions, sauce, Birds Eye	⅔ cup	17	4	13	90	5	0
Peppers, sweet (bell), green, raw	1 medium	8	2	6	32	1	0
Peppers, sweet (bell), red, raw	1 medium	8	2	6	32	1	0
Pepper stir-fry, Birds Eye	1 cup	5	1	4	25	1	0
Plantain, sliced	1 cup	48	4	44	179	1	0
Pumpkin, canned	1 cup	20	7	13	83	3	1
Potato, baked, skin	1 medium	37	4	33	161	4	0
Potato, baked, no skin	1 medium	34	2	32	145	3	0
Potato, boiled, no skin	1 medium	33	3	30	144	3	0
Potato, red-skinned, baked, skin	1 medium	34	3	31	154	4	0
Potato, russet, baked, skin	1 medium	37	4	33	168	5	0
Potato puffs	1 cup	39	4	35	284	4	14
Potatoes au gratin, mix, Betty Crocker	½ cup	23	1	22	150	3	6
Potatoes, cheesy scalloped, mix, Betty Crocker	½ cup	20	1	19	150	3	6
Potatoes, hash browns, frozen	½ cup	22	2	20	170	3	9

Food	Serving size	Carbohy-drates	Fiber	Net Carbs	Calories	Protein	Fat
Potatoes, hash browns, mix, Betty Crocker	½ cup	30	3	27	120	3	0
Potatoes, mashed	1 cup	35	4	31	223	4	9
Potatoes, mashed, from flakes	1 cup	32	5	27	237	4	12
Potatoes, mashed, from granules	1 cup	28	4	24	166	4	5
Potatoes, mashed, mix, Potato Buds	1 cup	38	2	36	320	6	16
Potatoes, scalloped	1 cup	26	5	21	211	14	18
Potatoes, scalloped, mix	½ cup	18	2	16	127	3	6
Potatoes, scalloped, Stouffer's	½ cup	18	0	18	140	6	5
Pumpkin, mashed	1 cup	12	3	9	49	2	0
Radicchio, raw, shredded	1 cup	2	0	2	9	1	0
Radish, oriental, raw	1 radish	14	5	9	61	2	0
Radish, red, raw, sliced	½ cup	2	1	1	12	0	0
Radish, white icicle, raw, sliced	½ cup	1	1	0	7	1	0
Rhubarb, raw	1 cup	6	2	4	26	1	0
Rhubarb, sweetened	1 cup	75	5	70	278	1	0
Roasted potatoes, broccoli, Birds Eye	⅔ cup	15	1	14	100	2	4
Rutabaga	1 cup	15	3	12	66	2	0

Food	Serving size	Carbohy-drates	Fiber	Net Carbs	Calories	Protein	Fat
Sauerkraut, canned	1 cup	6	4	2	27	1	0
Sauerkraut, packaged	1 cup	6	4	2	27	1	0
Scallions, raw	½ cup	4	2	2	16	1	0
Seven vegetable stir-fry, Birds Eye	1 cup	5	2	3	30	1	0
Snow peas	1 cup	11	5	6	67	5	0
Snow peas, raw	1 cup	5	2	3	26	2	0
Southwestern style corn, peppers, Green Giant	1 cup	24	1	23	120	4	1
Spaghetti squash	1 cup	10	2	8	42	1	0
Spinach, butter sauce, Green Giant	1 cup	8	4	4	70	4	2
Spinach, chopped	1 cup	10	6	4	54	6	0
Spinach, creamed, Stouffer's	½ cup	8	2	6	232	5	20
Spinach, raw, chopped	1 cup	1	1	0	7	1	0
Squash, summer	1 cup	8	3	5	36	2	1
Squash, summer, raw	1 cup	5	2	3	23	1	0
Sweet potato, baked, skin	1 medium	28	3	25	117	2	0
Sweet potato, canned, mashed	1 cup	60	4	56	358	5	0

Food	Serving size	Carbohy-drates	Fiber	Net Carbs	Calories	Protein	Fat
Sweet potato, canned, syrup	1 cup	50	6	44	212	3	1
Sweet potato, mashed, no skin	1 cup	80	6	72	344	5	1
Sweet potatoes, candied, Green Giant	1 cup	55	4	51	320	3	9
Szechuan vegetables, sesame sauce, Birds Eye	1 cup	9	2	7	60	1	2
Tater Tots, Ore-Ida	3 oz.	21	0	21	170	4	8
Tomato, cherry, raw	1 cup	7	2	5	31	1	0
Tomato paste	1 T	3	0	3	13	0	0
Tomato paste	6 oz. can	33	7	26	139	6	1
Tomato, plum, raw	1 medium	3	1	2	13	0	0
Tomato puree, canned	1 cup	24	5	19	100	4	0
Tomato, raw	1 medium	6	1	5	26	1	0
Tomato, raw, sliced	1 cup	6	1	5	26	1	0
Tomato, stewed, canned	1 cup	17	3	14	71	2	0
Tomato, sun-dried	½ cup	15	7	8	70	4	1
Tomato, sun-dried, olive oil	½ cup	13	3	10	117	3	8
Turnip	1 cup	8	3	5	33	1	0

Food	Serving size	Carbohy-drates	Fiber	Net Carbs	Calories	Protein	Fat
Turnip, mashed	1 cup	11	5	6	48	2	0
Turnip greens, chopped	1 cup	8	6	2	49	6	1
Turnip greens, raw, chopped	1 cup	3	2	1	15	1	0
Tuscan vegetables, herbed tomato sauce, Birds Eye	1 cup	7	2	5	50	1	2
Vegetables teriyaki, Green Giant	1 cup	5	2	3	64	2	4
Water chestnuts, sliced, canned	½ cup	9	2	7	35	1	0
Water chestnuts, sliced, raw	½ cup	9	2	7	35	1	0
Watercress, raw, chopped	1 cup	0	0	0	4	1	0
Winter blend vegetables, cheese sauce, Birds Eye	1⅓ cup	6	3	3	50	3	2
Winter squash, Birds Eye	½ cup	11	2	9	45	0	0
Yam, baked, skin	1 cup	38	5	33	158	2	0
Yellow snap beans	1 cup	10	4	6	44	2	0
Yellow snap beans, canned	1 cup	6	2	4	27	2	0
Zucchini, raw, sliced	1 cup	3	1	2	16	1	0
Zucchini, sliced	1 cup	7	3	4	29	1	0

YOGURT

High in protein, low in fat, and an excellent source of dietary calcium, yogurt is a favorite food for healthy eaters. At about 16 carbs per 8 ounces, however, even plain yogurt is on the high side for net carbs. Added fruit, flavorings, and sugar can add a *lot* more carbs. You don't have to give up your yogurt, though. Just choose brands that have the lowest carb counts, or try some of the reduced-carb products. (If you prefer soy yogurt, also known as cultured soy, see the section on soy foods in this book.)

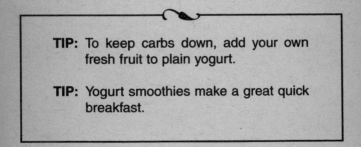

TIP: To keep carbs down, add your own fresh fruit to plain yogurt.

TIP: Yogurt smoothies make a great quick breakfast.

Food	Serving size	Carbohy-drates	Fiber	Net Carbs	Calories	Protein	Fat
Apple cobbler, Breyers	8 oz.	46	0	46	230	7	2
Black cherry, Breyers	8 oz.	46	0	46	240	9	2
Blueberry, Breyers	8 oz.	44	0	44	230	9	2
Custard style, fruit flavors, Yoplait	6 oz.	32	0	32	190	7	4
Light, fruit flavors, Yoplait	6 oz.	19	0	19	100	5	0
Light, Key lime pie, Breyers	8 oz.	11	0	11	60	4	0
Light, strawberry, Breyers	8 oz.	11	0	11	60	4	0
Low-fat, banana strawberry, Colombo	8 oz.	47	0	47	230	7	2
Fat-free, apricot mango, Stonyfield Farm	6 oz.	26	2	24	130	6	0
Fat-free, blueberry, Stonyfield Farm	6 oz.	26	2	24	130	6	0
Fat-free, Chocolate Underground, Stonyfield Farm	6 oz.	39	2	37	180	7	0
Fat-free, plain, Stonyfield Farm	6 oz.	14	2	12	80	8	0
Fat-free, raspberry, Stonyfield Farm	6 oz.	25	2	23	130	6	0
Frusion, banana berry blend	10 fl. oz.	52	0	52	270	8	4
Frusion, cherry berry blend	10 fl. oz.	53	0	53	280	8	4
Frusion, peach passion fruit	10 fl. oz.	51	0	51	270	8	4

Food	Serving size	Carbohy-drates	Fiber	Net Carbs	Calories	Protein	Fat
Frusion, strawberry kiwi blend	10 fl. oz.	52	0	52	270	8	4
Frusion, tropical fruit blend, Dannon	10 fl. oz.	52	0	52	270	8	4
Frusion, wild berry blend, Dannon	10 fl. oz.	53	0	53	280	8	4
Low-fat, Blueberries and Crème, Breyers	8 oz.	45	0	45	240	7	3
Low-fat, French vanilla, Colombo	8 oz.	32	0	32	180	8	3
Low-fat, fruit flavor	8 oz.	42	0	42	238	11	3
Low-fat, lemon, Colombo	8 oz.	32	0	32	180	8	2
Low-fat, Orange and Crème, Breyers	8 oz.	45	0	45	240	7	3
Low-fat, Peaches and Crème, Breyers	8 oz.	45	0	45	240	7	3
Low-fat, plain	8 oz.	16	0	16	143	12	4
Low-fat, plain, Colombo	8 oz.	16	0	16	130	10	3
Low-fat, plain, Dannon	8 oz.	18	0	18	150	12	4
Low-fat, Raspberries and Crème, Breyers	8 oz.	45	0	45	240	7	3
Low-fat, strawberry, Colombo	8 oz.	31	0	31	190	9	3
Low-fat, strawberry, Dannon	8 oz.	40	0	40	210	9	2
Low-fat, Strawberries and Crème, Breyers	8 oz.	45	0	45	240	7	3
Low-fat, vanilla, Colombo	8 oz.	32	0	32	180	8	2

Food	Serving size	Carbohy-drates	Fiber	Net Carbs	Calories	Protein	Fat
Low-fat, vanilla, Dannon	8 oz.	36	0	36	230	11	4
Low-fat, various flavors, Colombo	8 oz.	42	0	42	220	7	2
Mixed berry, Breyers	8 oz.	46	0	46	240	9	2
Nonfat, apple cinnamon, Breyers	8 oz.	22	0	22	120	8	0
Nonfat, French vanilla, Dannon	6 oz.	16	0	16	100	8	0
Nonfat, Key lime pie, Breyers	8 oz.	22	0	22	120	8	0
Nonfat, lemon chiffon, Breyers	8 oz.	21	0	21	120	8	0
Nonfat, plain	8 oz.	17	0	17	127	13	0
Nonfat, strawberry, Breyers	8 oz.	23	0	23	125	8	0
Nonfat, vanilla, Colombo	8 oz.	32	0	32	160	8	0
Nonfat, vanilla, Dannon	8 oz.	22	0	22	110	5	0
Peach, Breyers	8 oz.	45	0	45	230	9	2
Pineapple, Breyers	8 oz.	430	0	430	230	9	2
Raspberry, Breyers	8 oz.	46	0	46	240	9	2
Smoothie, Orange Crème, Breyers	10 fl. oz.	32	0	32	190	8	3
Smoothie, peach, Stonyfield Farm	10 fl. oz.	49	4	45	250	10	3
Smoothie, Peaches and Crème, Breyers	10 fl. oz.	32	0	32	190	8	3

Food	Serving size	Carbohy-drates	Fiber	Net Carbs	Calories	Protein	Fat
Smoothie, raspberry, Stonyfield Farm	10 fl. oz.	45	4	41	240	10	3
Smoothie, strawberry, Stonyfield Farm	10 fl. oz.	46	4	42	250	10	3
Smoothie, Strawberry Crème, Breyers	10 fl. oz.	32	0	32	190	8	3
Smoothie, Tropical Banana, Stonyfield Farm	10 fl. oz.	46	4	42	250	10	3
Smoothie, vanilla, Stonyfield Farm	10 fl. oz.	46	4	42	250	10	3
Smoothie, Wild Berry, Stonyfield Farm	10 fl. oz.	46	4	42	250	10	3
Strawberry, Breyers	8 oz.	46	0	46	240	9	2
Strawberry banana, Breyers	8 oz.	46	0	46	230	9	2
Vanilla, Breyers	8 oz.	46	0	46	230	7	2
Whole, plain	8 oz.	11	0	11	138	8	7

REDUCED-CARB PRODUCTS

Food	Serving size	Carbohy-drates	Fiber	Net Carbs	Calories	Protein	Fat
Carb Control, blueberries cream	4 oz.	3	0	3	60	5	3
Carb Control, peaches cream	4 oz.	3	0	3	60	5	3
Carb Control, raspberries cream	4 oz.	3	0	3	60	5	3
Carb Control, strawberry cream	4 oz.	3	0	3	60	5	3

Food	Serving size	Carbohy-drates	Fiber	Net Carbs	Calories	Protein	Fat
Carb Control, vanilla cream	4 oz.	3	0	3	60	5	3
Carb Countdown, blueberry	6 oz.	4	0	4	80	12	2
Carb Countdown, French vanilla	6 oz.	4	0	4	80	12	2
Carb Countdown, peach	6 oz.	4	0	4	80	12	2
Carb Countdown, raspberry	6 oz.	4	0	4	80	12	2
Carb Countdown, strawberry	6 oz.	4	0	4	80	12	2
Carb Countdown, strawberry banana	6 oz.	4	0	4	80	12	2
Carb Countdown smoothie, black cherry	10 fl. oz.	4	0	4	100	13	3
Carb Countdown smoothie, strawberry	10 fl. oz.	4	0	4	100	13	3
Carb Countdown smoothie, strawberry banana	10 fl. oz.	4	0	4	100	13	3

DR. ATKINS' NEW DIET REVOLUTION

The latest on the safety and effectiveness of the
Atkins approach

•

Dozens of new recipes and tips to jump-start weight loss

•

The amazing #1 bestseller that's helped millions!

by Robert C. Atkins, M.D.

0-06-001203-X•$7.99 US•$10.99 Can

ATK 0104